PROFESSIONALISM
in
MEDICAL ASSISTING

Kristiana D. Routh, RMA
Allied Health Consulting Services
Erie, Pennsylvania

PEARSON

Boston Columbus Indianapolis New York San Francisco Upper Saddle River
Amsterdam Cape Town Dubai London Madrid Milan Munich Paris Montréal Toronto
Delhi Mexico City São Paulo Sydney Hong Kong Seoul Singapore Taipei Tokyo

Publisher: Julie Levin Alexander
Publisher's Assistant: Regina Bruno
Editor-in-Chief: Marlene McHugh Pratt
Executive Editor: Joan Gill
Development Editor: Bronwen Glowacki
Editorial Assistant: Stephanie Kiel
Director of Marketing: David Gesell
Marketing Manager: Katrin Beacom
Senior Marketing Coordinator: Alicia Wozniak
Production Liaison: Pat Brown
Senior Media Editor: Matt Norris
Media Project Manager: Lorena Cerisano
Creative Director: Andrea Nix
Senior Art Director: Maria Guglielmo
Cover and Interior Designer: Christine Cantera
Cover Image: Minerva Studio/Shutterstock.com
Project Management/Compostion: Murugesh Rajkumar Namasivayam/PreMediaGlobal
Printing and Binding: R.R. Donnelley/Crawfordsville
Cover Printer: Lehigh-Phoenix Color/Hagerstown

Credits and acknowledgments for content borrowed from other sources and reproduced, with permission, in this book appear on appropriate page within text.

Library of Congress Cataloging-in-Publication Data
Routh, Kristiana Sue.
　　Professionalism in medical assisting / Kristiana Sue Routh.
　　　　p. ; cm.
　　Includes index.
　　ISBN-13: 978-0-13-254546-4
　　ISBN-10: 0-13-254546-2
　　I. Title.
　　[DNLM: 1. Allied Health Personnel. 2. Professional Competence. 3. Professional Role. W 21.5]
　　610.73'7069—dc23

2012036339

10 9 8 7 6 5 4 3 2 1

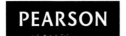

ISBN 10: 0-13-254546-2
ISBN 13: 978-0-13-254546-4

Brief Contents

Detailed Contents

To my husband and best friend, Jeremy, for his unwavering love, support, and strength. You are the best gift I have ever been given.

To my daughter Kaley Tailor, I will always love you beyond the universe. Remember to dream big and be confident—you can move mountains.

To my mother for believing in me and making me the woman I am today and to my father for teaching me the value of confidence and respect—mi manchi ogni giorno.

This book has been written to provide students with a competitive edge in the field of medical assisting. Some areas of the United States will see job fields saturated with both experienced and newly graduated medical assistants. What will set apart one equally trained and credentialed medical assistant from another? I believe the answer is professionalism. Employers are searching for people who are able to work cohesively with others, who treat all patients with respect and kindness, and who have a moral and ethical compass directing their actions.

This text has been written in a clear, easy-to-read manner. The chapters are organized to flow in succession for the medical assistant preparing to complete his or her classroom training, progressing into the externship, and then the graduate's entry into the actual field of medical assisting. Careful consideration has gone into the creation of the case studies and role-play scenarios. These will help the reader develop critical thinking skills and create professional responses to the situations given.

Medical assistants who read this text and put it into action will not only stand out because of their professional behavior but will also have a competitive edge for advancement throughout their career.

Kristiana Routh is a registered medical assistant who has worked primarily in the field of clinical medical assisting early in her career. She began teaching in the Medical Assisting program at Tri-State Business Institute, now Fortis Institute, in Erie, Pennsylvania. During her years of teaching, she realized her love and passion for educating students through real-life applications, challenging and thought-provoking activities, and competency-based learning. Today, she is the owner of Allied Health Consulting Services. She provides consulting services to educational facilities regarding curriculum development. She also works directly with physicians and dentists as a practice management consultant. She has written a variety of health-related articles for Internet publications.

Kristiana lives with her husband and daughter in Girard, Pennsylvania, near beautiful Lake Erie.

Acknowledgments

I deeply appreciate the invaluable editorial advice and direction provided by the following educators and healthcare professionals:

Stacey Ashford AAS, CPC
Instructor
Remington College
Cleveland, Ohio

Norma Bird, MEd, BS, CMA (AAMA)
Medical Assisting Program
    Coordinator
Idaho State University
Pocatello, Indiana

Chrystal Gaunt, CMA (AAMA)
Medical Assisting Instructor
Carrington College
Spokane, Washington

Cheri Goretti, MA, MT (ASCP), CMA (AAMA)
Professor and Director, Medical
    Assisting and Allied Health
    Programs
Quinebaug Valley Community
    College
Danielson, Connecticut

Jennifer Holmes, BA
Curriculum Development
    Specialist
Concorde Career Colleges, Inc.
Mission, Kansas

Diane Morlock, MS, CMA (AAMA)
Medical Assisting Coordinator
Owens Community College
Toledo, Ohio

Lisa Nagle, CMA (AAMA) BSEd
Program Director
Augusta Technical College
Augusta, Georgia

Martha L. Olah, RN
Allied Health Instructor
Remington College, Cleveland
    West Campus
North Olmsted, Ohio

Kathleen M. Olewinski, MS, RHIA, NHA, FACHE
Program Director
Bryant & Stratton College—
    Milwaukee Market
Milwaukee, Wisconsin

Lynn Slack, BS, CMA (AAMA)
Medical Programs Director
Kaplan Career Institute
Pittsburgh, Pennsylvania

Antoinette Woodall, BA, CMA, CMRS, MD
Remington College, Cleveland
    West Campus
North Olmsted, Ohio

Lisa Wright CMA (AAMA), MT (ASCP), SH
Medical Assisting Program
    Coordinator, Medical Support
    Programs Department Chair
Bristol Community College
Falls River, Massachusetts

Patti Zint, CMAA, AHI
Program Director, Medical
    Assisting/Healthcare
    Administration
Carrington College
Phoenix, Arizona

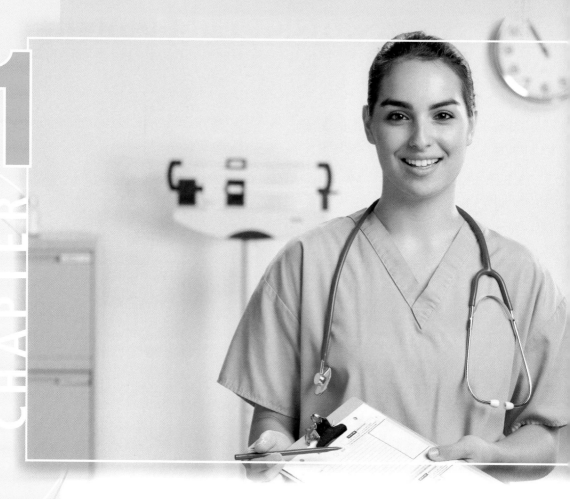

CHAPTER 1

Professionalism as a Student

LEARNING OBJECTIVES

- Explain how morals and ethics relate to professionalism.

- Outline why the externship is a vital component to forming professional traits within the student.

- Explain why an educational skills résumé would be used by a new graduate.

- Name six components that should be included in all résumés.

- Describe why cover letters are specifically tailored for each prospective job.

- List four of the six ways to project a positive self-image when interviewing for a position.

- Identify four of the five things to avoid when interviewing for a job.

KEY TERMS
cover letter
ethics
initiative
morals
organic
portfolio
professionalism
punctual
résumé
syllabus

Workplace Scenario

Emma Lawson is in her final term of school and will be graduating in three weeks. She has been on externship for the past four weeks at Smithfield Regional OB-GYN Associates. Here, Emma has had the opportunity to work in both the administrative and clinical areas; when given the choice, she chooses to work in the clinical area. Elaine, the office manager, has just called Emma into the office to discuss how Emma has been progressing through the externship. During their discussion, Elaine asks Emma if she would like to schedule a formal interview for a new position to assist a new doctor who is joining the practice.

Introduction

Professionalism as it relates to this text refers to one's behavior, excellence at interaction with others, and a poised and self-assured manner in which one carries oneself. Students may not realize that the opportunity to develop qualities of sound professionalism begins right inside the classroom. This chapter will help you explore the manner in which you as a student can strive to cultivate positive behaviors and professional qualities.

The Beginnings of a Professional Student

Instructors and educators are often the first individuals to notice a student's quality of professionalism. From the very first class of a medical assistant's training, instructors are looking for students who are committed, eager, and motivated to learn. Although there are many characteristics that embody students with a great sense of professionalism, they are not immediately identified in all students.

Cultivating a Professional Image

Every student should work to create a professional image that is unique to the individual. Although there are major overlying concepts that deal with professionalism, such as character traits that will be discussed later in the text, there are also personal aspects that will help shape and mold the student's perception of professionalism.

Ethics and Morals

Morals refer to what one believes to be right, true, and honorable. **Ethics** refers to one's moral conduct, or the way in which one practices his or her moral beliefs. *Medical ethics* refers to moral customs and principles relating to healthcare. Box 1-1 displays the Code of Ethics of the American Association of Medical Assistants; many medical assistant textbooks discuss medical ethics in more detail. Morals and ethics are shaped by a variety of factors including religious beliefs, culture, race, and socioeconomic and demographic factors. When defining a professional image, personal ethics and morals will help the student develop his or her own perception of

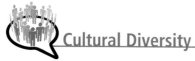 Cultural Diversity

The classroom is a perfect learning opportunity for acceptance of various cultural beliefs and morals. The cultural backgrounds of students in a particular school can vary quite significantly. As the medical assistant student looks ahead to working in the culturally diverse field of healthcare, he or she can take the opportunity to learn about cultural interactions from peers while in the classroom. This is an invaluable learning tool to prepare for the workplace.

BOX 1-1 Code of Ethics of the American Association of Medical Assistants

PREAMBLE

The Code of Ethics of AAMA shall set forth principles of ethical and moral conduct as they relate to the medical profession and the particular practice of medical assisting.

Members of the AAMA dedicated to the conscientious pursuit of their profession, and thus desiring to merit the high regard of the entire medical profession and the respect of the general public which they serve, do hereby pledge themselves to strive always to:

Human Dignity

I. Render service with full respect for the dignity of humanity;

Confidentiality

II. Respect confidential information obtained through employment unless legally authorized or required by responsible performance of duty to divulge such information;

Honor

III. Uphold the honor and high principles of the profession and accept its disciplines;

Continued Study

IV. Seek to continually improve the knowledge and skills of medical assistants for the benefit of patients and professional colleagues;

Responsibility for Improved Community

V. Participate in additional service activities aimed toward improving the health and well-being of the community.

Copyright by the American Association of Medical Assistants, Inc. Reprinted with permission

professionalism. While morals and ethics are considered **organic**, or found within the person, character traits are a learned behavior (■ Figure 1-1). These will be discussed next.

Character Traits

Carrying oneself in a professional manner may come very easy to some and prove to be more of a struggle for others. In general, many of the traits of a professional student are brought to life during the first day of class when an instructor reads the **syllabus**, outlining the course-work, assignments, and expectations of the student. How students carry out what is expected of them will begin to develop and shape their views of professionalism, even though they may not be

■ FIGURE 1-1

Morals, ethics, and character traits help develop one's sense of professionalism.

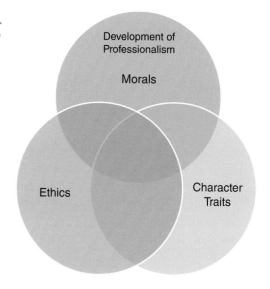

aware it is even happening. The following is a list of traits demonstrated by a student portraying professionalism in the classroom setting:

- Good attendance
- Punctuality
- Being prepared
- Displaying responsibility
- Accepting responsibility
- Doing a thorough job
- Maintaining excellent personal hygiene and appearance
- Demonstrating respect for others
- Showing initiative
- Creating personal boundaries

With consistent practice and training on these traits, students will be well on their way to a successful start to a professional career. Let us take a closer look at each of these traits.

ATTENDANCE Attendance is one of the most important components to a student's education and professional development. A professional student is always in class with the exception of an illness or an extenuating situation, such as jury duty. In instances of absence, a physician's excuse or other documentation is provided when the student returns. Many medical assistant courses involve heavy course-work and missing even one class may place a student behind peers. Also, many students do not consider the fact that their school attendance is often a deciding factor for externship placement as well as employment.

PUNCTUALITY A **punctual** student shows professionalism by arriving early to class. Students should arrive at least five minutes before the designated start time, allowing them to get situated and prepared for the day's lesson. Punctuality not only shows professionalism as a character trait but also demonstrates a respect for the instructor's—and other students'—time.

PREPAREDNESS As a student in the classroom, being prepared is demonstrated by having all materials open and ready for use in class, including pens, notebooks, and textbooks. Cell phones should be turned off and put away. The ring of a cell phone can be a major distraction during instruction and learning.

Career Tips

Cell phones have begun to gain popularity and, in some cases, acceptance in the workplace or classroom setting. If a cell phone is permitted to be turned on while you are at work or in class, consider keeping the phone on vibration mode as not to cause unnecessary distraction. Also, consider the ring tone. Current songs, funny voices, and overly melodic tunes are not viewed as appropriate ring tones for a professional.

RESPONSIBILITY There are two components that comprise the trait of responsibility. First, a student practicing and learning in the classroom will *want* to display responsibility. *Displaying* responsibility is done through timely completion of assignments, doing something when first asked, and taking care of personal and school property. *Accepting* responsibility is often a much more advanced character trait. A true professional will accept responsibility for his or her errors, such as not completing a task that was assigned or simply forgetting all together to complete a task. It is unfortunate that many make excuses or try to blame others to simply make themselves look or feel better. However, it is honesty coupled with responsibility that builds character. This is what instructors, educators, mentors, and employers are striving to find.

BEING THOROUGH New students, already having busy schedules, may find their coursework responsibilities difficult to work into their already busy day-to-day lives. Often, students, along with their new course-work, have full- or part-time jobs, families to take care of, and other commitments outside of the classroom. Attitudes toward homework and other assignments often are lackluster and students want to complete assignments as quickly as possible. True learning comes from careful reading, concentrated thought, and well-thought-out reasoning. Being thorough in homework and assignments will show instructors that you are serious about your learning, and in turn serious about your up-and-coming profession.

PERSONAL HYGIENE AND APPEARANCE A student must take personal hygiene and appearance into consideration when evaluating his or her own professional image. Students should bathe and brush their teeth every day. Hair should be neatly styled and antiperspirant should be used daily. Uniforms should be clean and pressed. If uniforms are not mandated, the clothing you wear should be respectable and modest. Offensive language or suggestive slogans on clothing along with shorts and tank tops should be avoided. Shoes should be comfortable and have a slip-resistant sole.

DEMONSTRATING RESPECT FOR OTHERS Respecting others is often something that is learned by observation starting as a young child. Students who find respecting others challenging may have lacked a positive role model earlier in their life. Disrespect is *never* appropriate; such

■ TABLE 1-1 **Demonstrating Respect for Others**

Respectful Actions

• Arriving on time for class, work, and other appointments

• Not speaking over others, waiting for your turn to talk

• Listening to another point of view and *not* passing judgment

• Helping someone who is in need

• Maintaining a person's privacy

• Not participating in gossip

• Maintaining composure during an argument or altercation

• Refraining from using foul or inappropriate language

students may need to work on nurturing this particular character trait. ■ Table 1-1 lists ways students can practice demonstrating respect for others.

SHOWING INITIATIVE **Initiative** is considered doing more than what is expected, being resourceful and creative, and tackling issues with ingenuity without having to be told. This is a highly valuable trait of professionalism within the workforce, and it often will be a key characteristic of those who are promoted for more advanced jobs. As a student, initiative can be displayed by reading ahead on assignments, staying after class to practice competencies, helping tutor other students, or attempting to create new studying methods.

CREATING PERSONAL BOUNDARIES Successful integration of work and personal lives is important for those in the workforce. A common downfall of many is their inability to separate personal life from work life. For example, employees will bring their problems from home to work and discuss these problems with coworkers. This will ultimately lead to drama within the office as personal matters are fuel for gossip and lead to a loss of production within the office. Students should take the opportunity to begin practicing setting personal boundaries while in the classroom. Measures should be taken if habits of discussing personal problems have already been formed.

Professionalism from Class to Externship

Students should begin to implement actions of professionalism throughout their course-work while learning to become a medical assistant. The character traits mentioned earlier along with the student's personal and moral ethics should begin to form a well-rounded professional.

Difficulties in Class

The true "color" or nature of a student's professional behavior will come under scrutiny when the student is faced with a difficulty or challenge. Students may face challenges within the classroom as they tackle difficult assignments, work with challenging instructors, or deal with troublesome classmates. Again, these situations should all be viewed as learning opportunities from which the student can learn and apply the knowledge gained to handle challenges that may arise within the workforce while on the job later down the road.

Preparing for Externship

Thoughts of externship will begin to surface for students as they near the end of their formal classroom trainings and practicum. Externship is an exciting learning opportunity for medical assistant students as this will often be the first time the student will experience working within the actual healthcare field. It is during the externship that the student's professionalism will be closely monitored, critiqued, and graded. Some students fail to recognize the sheer importance of the externship experience. The externship should be thought of as a continual job interview. As such, most externship sites will require students to complete an interview before being accepted as an extern. This interview must not be taken lightly, and preparation is essential.

DEVELOPING A RÉSUMÉ The first task, when preparing for externship, is to develop a **résumé**. A résumé is a summary of credentials, work history, experience, training, and education. A well-thought-out and carefully developed résumé is going to be one of the student's most valuable tools as the student prepares to enter the job market. There are two main types of résumé formats: the chronological format and the educational skills format. With a chronological résumé, events and credentials are placed in the order of their occurrence starting with the most recent first. Therefore, new graduates without much work experience will find the educational skills résumé more useful. ■ Table 1-2 highlights dos and don'ts for résumé creation. ■ Figures 1-2 and 1-3 show the chronological and educational skills formats.

Regardless of the résumé format, there are core components that must be present in all résumés. These items include the following:

1. **Heading:** Your name, address, email address, and telephone number are included at the very top of the résumé. Generally, this information is printed in a larger font and often boldfaced.
2. **Objective:** This states your goal, which you want to achieve. Objectives should be concise and clearly written.
3. **Education:** Schooling and training are generally written in reverse chronological order. Externship and practicum should be listed immediately after for new or recent graduates. Workshops, conferences, and additional trainings can also be listed here.

■ TABLE 1-2 **Dos and Don'ts of Creating a Résumé**

Do	Don't
Highlight all your marketable skills.	Exaggerate or lie about skills you are lacking.
Spend time working on your résumé.	Complete the résumé just to "get it done."
Use a standard résumé format or template; many of these can be found for free on the Internet.	Try to create your own style; employers want to see a professional and polished résumé.
Proofread, checking for spelling and grammar errors.	Send out your résumé without having at least two people read it and provide honest critique.
Print on high-quality résumé paper.	Print it on copy paper or brightly colored paper.
Backup your résumé to an external device, for example, a USB drive.	Delete or get rid of your résumé as soon as it is printed; résumés will always need to be updated.

HECTOR GUTTIEREZ, RMA

8 LOCK DRIVE NEW YORK, NY
(123)555-4141
HECTORG@ANYWHERE.COM

OBJECTIVE: To begin a rewarding career as a clinical medical assistant.

PROFESSIONAL ORGANIZATIONS AND CREDENTIALS

- Registered Medical Assistant through American Medical Technologists
- CPR Certified by the American Red Cross
- Member of the American Association of Medical Assistants

PROFESSIONAL EXPERIENCE

2007–Present Clinical Medical Assistant, Hayfield Internal Medicine, New York, NY
I perform clinical duties including obtaining vital signs, perform phlebotomy, administer shots and vaccinations, and assist with minor in-office surgical procedures.
05/05–02/07 Medical Assistant, Jefferson Regional Medical Center, Pittsburgh, PA
I worked in the admissions office registering new hospital patients, scheduling appointments, and creating patient statements.
08/00–04/05 Medical Assistant, Preferred Primary Care Physicians, Pittsburgh, PA
I worked as a clinical and administrative medical assistant. I worked all aspects of the medical office from scheduling, filing and billing to obtaining vitals, performing EKGs, and scheduling out-patient testing.

EDUCATION

Erie Business Center—Erie, PA
Associates in Specialized Business, Medical Assisting, 2000

REFERENCES

Available upon request

■ FIGURE 1-2

A résumé using the chronological format.

Priysha Kaur-Ali

3200 State Street, Sheldon, PA 12345
555-814-1230
pka@anywhere.com

Objective

To obtain a challenging career in the field of medical assisting.

Training and Skills

I learned to competently complete the following skills with a grade of 90% or higher:

CLINICAL SKILLS

- Obtain vital signs including height, weight, blood pressure, pulse, respirations, and pulse oximetry
- Perform venipuncture, including use of the butterfly needle
- Collect urine samples
- Perform EKGs
- Administer intramuscular, subcutaneous, and intradermal injections

ADMINSITRATIVE SKILLS

- Understand and schedule various appointment methods
- Perform CPT and ICD-10 coding
- Create new patient files
- Copy, scan, and fax documents
- Sort and annotate mail

CPR Certified- American Heart Association, December 2012

Education

2010–2012 Sheldon Community College Sheldon, PA

Associates Degree in Specialized Business- Medical Assisting
   Graduated with honors, GPA 3.7

2006–2010 Sheldon Area High School Sheldon, PA
High School Diploma
   Graduated with honors, GPA 3.5

References

References are available on request.

■ FIGURE 1-3

A résumé using the educational skills format.

4. **Credentials:** Information about professional credentials, such as CMA (AAMA) certification or RMA (AMT)/registration, is included. If you do not have any credentials, do not include this section on your résumé.

5. **Employment:** Work experience is also listed in reverse chronological order, your most recent job set first. Include a brief description of duties and responsibilities you held with each job.

6. **References:** The reference section should always state "Available upon request" or "Furnished upon request." It is not appropriate to include the name, telephone number, or address of references you will be using.

Memberships and affiliations with professional organizations are also important to include in a résumé. In fact, becoming a member of an organization adds value to one's professionalism. Members of professional medical organizations will often receive periodicals and newsletter updates that contain information regarding trends in healthcare, opportunities for continuing education, and advances in medical technologies. All students should seriously consider sitting for certification examinations for which they are qualified. The certified medical assistant (CMA) is a test taken through the American Association of Medical Assistants (AAMA). And the registered medical assistant (RMA) credential is offered through American Medical Technologists (AMT). It is recommended that all medical assistants become members of the AAMA, even if they are unable to sit for certification for the CMA (AAMA) exam (■ Figure 1-4).

Cover Letters

A **cover letter** (■ Figure 1-5) is a letter of introduction that accompanies a résumé. Nearly all job applications require a cover letter. Cover letters should be brief and to the point—stating the purpose of the letter and explaining why you are a good candidate for the job position. Cover letters, unlike résumés, must be custom written for each prospective employer or externship site, and contact information should be included. Some job advertisements request that the applicant include a salary request. Only reference a salary range if the job advertisement specifically requests one, and even then it is best you include a notation that indicates that the salary range is negotiable. Proofreading is exceptionally important when creating a cover letter as prospective employees will be critiquing the content of the letter. Always have someone else proofread the cover letter, as others will often find mistakes we tend to miss ourselves. ■ Table 1-3 lists pitfalls and things to avoid when creating a cover letter.

■ **FIGURE 1-4**

Becoming a member of the American Association of Medical Assistants shows commitment to your profession. Reprinted with permission from American Association of Medical Assistants, Chicago, IL. © American Association of Medical Assistants.

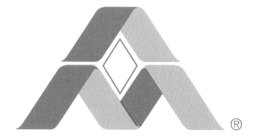

Ralph Taylor
222 East Main St.
Chicago, IL 60601
(312) 555-1212

May 20, 20XX

James Stark, M.D.
1450 N. Devonshire
Chicago, IL 60611

Dear Dr. Stark:

This letter is in response to your recent advertisement in the May 19, 20XX, <u>Chicago Sun News</u> for a certified medical assistant.

I believe that my qualifications are a good match for your position. During my medical assisting program at Central State College in Hometown, Illinois, I maintained a 3.6 GPA on a 4.0 scale.

My medical assisting program at Central State College was completed in December 20XX. I passed the American Association of Medical Assistants' certification examination January 27, 20XX. Currently I am completing an associate degree program at CSC and plan to graduate in June 20XX.

The enclosed résumé includes my experience as a part-time nursing assistant for Dr. Jane Young in her family practice office.

I look forward to meeting you to discuss your position needs and my qualifications.

Thank you for your consideration.

Sincerely,

Ralph Taylor

Ralph Taylor, CMA (AAMA)

■ FIGURE 1-5

An example of a well-written cover letter.

Developing a Portfolio

A **portfolio** is a collection of documents that shows the aptitude and accomplishments of the student or job candidate. A portfolio is often created in a three-ring binder or a specially designed portfolio system. The first page of each portfolio should be a copy of the résumé. Additional items in a portfolio include the following:

- A photocopy of any degrees that have been obtained
- A letter of recommendation from your externship site coordinator after completion of the externship

■ TABLE 1-3 **Cover Letter Pitfalls**

Common Mistakes

• Not addressing the cover letter to a specific person in the company or organization. Be sure to check the name for title and correct spelling.

• Failing to clearly state the position for which you are applying.

• Sending a cover letter that is too long. One-page letters work best.

• Sending a letter that is poorly worded or has spelling or typing errors.

• Not including your own contact information.

- Copies of certification cards, such as CPR and credentials
- Copies of any professional licenses
- Copies of awards and certificates

A student preparing for externship should also include graded copies of competencies that demonstrate knowledge of learned skills. The portfolio is then taken along to interviews and shown to the prospective employers. Some employers may ask for copies of the documents to be added to the application file.

Preparing for the Interview

You have created the résumé, cover letter, and portfolio. Now, it is necessary to focus on interviewing for an externship or a job within the field. Practicing interviewing with a friend is an extremely helpful tool and can target specific interview questions that may cause one to slip up. Box 1-2 lists common questions asked during an interview and can be used for practice. Being confident with your answers while not mistaking confidence for arrogance is vital. The difference between confidence and arrogance will be discussed in Chapter 2; however, here is an example to show the difference:

> *While at an interview for externship, Rosa is asked about her strengths. Rosa's confident answer might be, "I have been told that I am a fast learner. I know that will help when I begin working*

BOX 1-2 Practice Interview Questions

- What are your strengths?
- What are your weaknesses?
- What has been your favorite job? Why?
- What are your goals for the next year, for the next five years?
- Why do you want to work for this company?
- Why should I hire you?
- What are your qualifications?
- What has been one of your biggest accomplishments?
- How did you handle a difficult situation in the past that had a positive outcome?

because I won't slow down those who are training me." However, this same sentiment told in arrogance might sound like this: "I am really smart and everything always comes quickly to me. I just hope I won't get bored."

The externship interview does not end with the interviewer asking the candidate questions. Many times the candidate has the opportunity to ask questions of the interviewer regarding the organization and the position. These questions should be thoughtfully considered as they are an extension of the interviewing process. The following questions are not only appropriate to ask during an externship interview but also a prospective job interview:

- How would you describe a typical work day?
- What challenges would someone in this position face?
- What are the expectations of a person holding this job position?

ARE THERE GROWTH AND CAREER OPPORTUNITIES AVAILABLE? A POSITIVE IMAGE In addition to poise and confidence, a positive image will go a long way during a job interview. Portray a positive image by following these simple rules:

- When sitting across from your prospective employer, do not sit with your legs crossed at the knee or have your arms draped over the back of a chair. While it is important to look comfortable, it would be more appropriate to sit with both feet planted firmly on the ground and hands crossed gently in your lap (■ Figure 1-6).
- Remember to speak and breathe slowly. Nerves can sometimes cause one to speak and breathe rapidly.

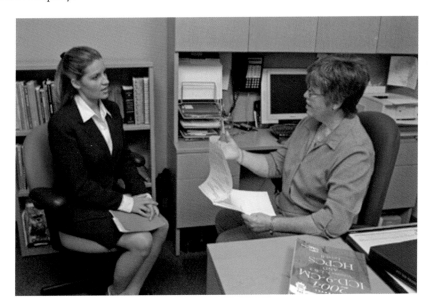

■ **FIGURE 1-6**

A medical assistant should display a positive appearance during the interview.

Source: Michal Heron/Pearson Education.

- It is nice to close an interview by saying something similar to "Thank you very much for the chance you have given me to interview for this position. I look forward to hearing from you with your response."
- Always arrive at least fifteen minutes before your scheduled appointment time. Showing up right on time or late shows a lack of respect for the interviewer's time.
- Prepare a list of questions to ask the interviewer. Far too often, those who are being interviewed do not ask questions about the job. Asking questions shows a sincere desire and initiative.
- Do not plan to discuss pay scale or salary during the initial interview, unless it is brought up by the interviewer. To do otherwise does not show tact.

THINGS TO AVOID When preparing for an interview there are a few things to keep in mind. Many of these ideas could be considered common sense; however, it does not stop individuals from showing up to interviews for jobs or externships looking far from professional. Consider these pieces of advice:

- **Wear conservative and muted colors during your interview.** While it is important to be able to express yourself, loud and bold colors can be a distraction to a possible new employer.
- **Consider modesty.** For women, it is important to look professional by not wearing tight pants, short skirts, or low-cut tops. Also, wear sensible footwear. High heels, rubber clogs, sneakers, and open-toe shoes should be changed to a more professional style of shoe. Men should not wear shorts or ill-fitting pants. Dress slacks, a button-up shirt, and tie should be worn. Business coats and suits are also acceptable. Men should wear sensible dress shoes and avoid sneakers and clogs.
- **Cover up your tattoos.** If you have tattoos on your arms or legs, consider covering them for the interview. If you have a tattoo on the torso or forearms that might be visible while wearing a uniform, ask the employer about their policies regarding tattoos. It may be necessary to find alternate means of covering up, when policies dictate.
- **Remove the body piercings.** If there are more than three piercings in your ears, or piercings on your face, consider removing them for the interview. Once again, it is important to find out the policy of the organization regarding body piercings. If you cannot remove the piercing for an extended period of time, purchase a clear or flesh colored piece of jewelry or retainer to lessen the visibility of the piercing. In some instances, it may be required to permanently remove the piercing. If this is something that you are not comfortable with, you should not consider taking the job if it is offered.
- **Consider the language used.** It is never appropriate to use off-color or foul language in a workplace, let alone during a job interview. If foul language is a part of your daily social life, it is important to keep it at home and to make a more presentable and professional image for yourself in the working world.

After Externship

Completing the externship phase of training is an extremely rewarding achievement. In some cases, students have excelled at the externship site and have been offered employment. Other times, even though a student may have excelled, the site may not have had job openings available. In this case, the new graduate will begin to embark in the process of finding a job within the field. Though finding a job can be difficult, it is imperative that one does not give up and continue to apply for jobs that are of interest.

END OF CHAPTER REVIEW

LEARNING OBJECTIVE REVIEW

Complete each learning objective to the best of your ability.

1. Explain how morals and ethics relate to professionalism.

   _____

   _____

   _____

   _____

   _____

2. Outline why the externship is a vital component to forming professional traits within the student.

   _____

   _____

   _____

   _____

   _____

3. Clarify why an educational skills résumé would be used by a new graduate.

   _____

   _____

   _____

   _____

   _____

4. Name six components that should be included in all résumés.

   _____

   _____

   _____

   _____

   _____

5. Describe why cover letters are specifically tailored for each prospective job.

_____

_____

_____

_____

_____

6. List four of the six ways to project a positive self-image when interviewing for a position.

_____

_____

_____

_____

_____

7. Identify four of the five things to avoid when interviewing for a job.

_____

_____

_____

_____

_____

KEY TERMS

Use each of the following key terms in a sentence that demonstrates your understanding of the word.

1. cover letter: _____

_____

2. ethics:_____

_____

3. initiative:_____

_____

4. morals:_____

_____

5. organic:_____

_____

6. portfolio:_____

_____

7. professionalism:_____

_____

8. punctual:_____

_____

9. résumé:_____

_____

10. syllabus:_____

_____

CRITICAL THINKING

Reread the workplace scenario at the beginning of the chapter and answer the following questions.

1. Emma eagerly accepts the opportunity to schedule an interview. Elaine asks Emma to bring a portfolio to the interview to share with the new doctor. Emma is nervous because she does not have a portfolio ready. She is not sure what she should include, but she certainly wants to highlight that during her schooling she had only missed two days of school. *What do you think Emma should include in her portfolio? How could she bring attention to her near perfect attendance record?*

_____

_____

_____

_____

_____

2. During the interview Emma is told that though the new doctor she will be working for does not perform abortions, he often treats women who have had or are planning on having an abortion. Elaine further explains to Emma the importance that professionalism plays when dealing with such sensitive matters and how all employees must be able to maintain the highest level of professionalism, regardless of the employee's personal views. *Explain how Emma's morals and ethics would play a role in her decision to accept this position.*

_____

_____

_____

_____

_____

3. Emma has heard from some of the employees at the office that they are not paid as much as other medical assistants at other specialty offices; however, the benefits are outstanding. *Emma wants to discuss this with Elaine but is not sure how to address the issue tactfully. What should Emma do?*

_____

_____

_____

_____

_____

DO IT YOURSELF!

Complete the modules below to demonstrate your understanding of the chapter.

Module A

Review the résumé on the following page. Proofread for errors and list the changes that must be made before it is sent out to a prospective employer.

Sheila Smallman, RMA

6223 West 14th Avenue,
Albany, NY,
sheilasmalls@ANYWHERE.COM

OBJECTIVE:
To begin a rewarding career as a clinical medical assistant.

Professional Credentials

- Registered Medcial Assistant, American Medical Technologies
- CPR Certfied

Wirk Experience

Jan. 2012- May 2012 Medical Assistant Extern, Albany Internal Medicine,
   Albany, NY
April 2009- Current Cashier, Whole-Foods Market, Albay, NY

Education

Albany community colege
Associates in Specialized Business, Medical Assisting, Graduated June 2012
Essex County High School
High School Diploma, Graduated June 2011

References

Joan Emmerson (Instructor) Albany Community College (111) 555-7896

Module B

Provide two unique examples of ways a student or extern could demonstrate each of the following character traits:

1. Good attendance

   _____

   _____

2. Punctuality

   _____

   _____

3. Being prepared

   _____

   _____

4. Displaying responsibility

   _____

   _____

5. Accepting responsibility

   _____

   _____

6. Doing a thorough job

   _____

   _____

7. Maintaining excellent personal hygiene and appearance

   _____

   _____

8. Demonstrating respect for others

   _____

   _____

9. Showing initiative

   _____

   _____

10. Creating personal boundaries

   _____

   _____

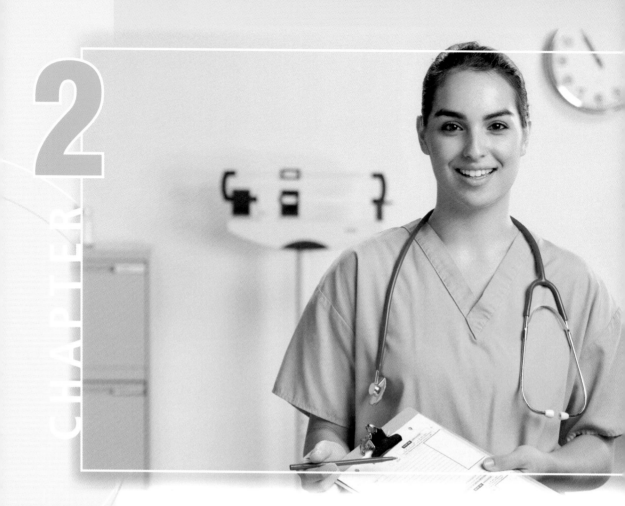

Professionalism on the Job

LEARNING OBJECTIVES

- Explain the importance of understanding a personal skill set.
- Identify why it is important to recognize personal limitations when applying for a job.
- List and describe four of the five resources that are helpful when beginning a job search.
- Describe the difference between confidence and arrogance.
- Explain the duties of a mentor.

KEY TERMS

arrogance

competence

confidence

mentor

networking

parameters

role model

skill set

staffing agency

temporary job

temp-to-hire

Workplace Scenario

Sue Ellen Ferrier has just finished her externship for medical assisting. She will be graduating in three weeks. She applied for a help-wanted ad that stated "P/T Clinical Medical Assistant needed for fast-paced pediatric office. Entry-level position, but some experience preferred." Sue Ellen's interview is at 3 pm/tomorrow.

Introduction

Welcome to the field of medical assisting. Understanding the skills and responsibilities medical assistants have in this field is an important step in being a successful medical office team member. The information and concepts presented in this chapter are designed to get the medical assistant's new career started on the right foot. As a student learning in the classroom, this book will help you gain an on-the-job perspective from a vantage point. The things you learn in this and the following chapters will help you prepare for a successful externship and career.

Starting Off on the Right Foot

Medical assisting can be a very rewarding and successful career. By the end of a medical assistant training program, many students will have felt the pressure of learning the intricacies of the human body, performing and applying the knowledge obtained through competencies, and facing the challenges of working in the field through externship experiences. It is important to realize the high demand in the field for medical assisting as well as the stiff competition that exists for coveted and desired positions.

Obtaining a position in the field of medical assisting is a task that must be pursued with knowledge, confidence, and skill. New graduates often will use the first few years after their schooling to explore various options and settings within the field of medical assisting. Some graduates will accept the very first position they are offered, only to find out later down the road that they are not a good fit for the position. Others may turn down a position because they simply did not like learning about it in school. As a new medical assistant, you should enter the job force with unbiased opinions and excitement. It is very important that you understand the strengths and weaknesses that you possess as a person and identify your personal **skill set** or specific areas of medical assisting in which you excel and you enjoy; these tasks are key to finding your right fit within the field.

Role Models

Identifying a role model is especially important when the hopes of success are high when beginning a new career in life. A **role model** is someone whom you hold in high esteem based on the way the role model lives out his or her personal and professional life, often demonstrating honesty, integrity, and self-discipline. Role models will demonstrate how to overcome obstacles that we face in life, obstacles that may arise out of one's environment or personal choices that one makes. Booker T. Washington, an influential educator and author, explained success best when he said, "Success is to be measured not so much by the position that one has reached in life as by the obstacles which he has overcome."[1]

Many people look to family members as their role models: parents, grandparents, aunts, uncles, or siblings. Others may not have a strong family background and may be discouraged

---

[1]http://www.brainyquote.com/quotes/authors/b/booker_t_washington.html#2VT1T0J8j0IKuOT2.99 (accessed July 21, 2012).

by this. When strong family role models are not present in your life you may choose to look to instructors, employers, coworkers, and friends to serve as positive examples for a successful life.

The Job Search

Graduates are exceptionally excited to be able to search for a job and begin their career as medical assistants. Chapter 1 outlined how to create effective résumés and cover letters. Now, it is important discuss how to successfully begin a job search.

Determining Your Needs and Limitations

You will undoubtedly search through dozens of job ads through various media: newspaper, Internet, local employment agencies. Understanding your needs and your limitations is very important applying for a position. Consider the following questions:

- Am I willing to relocate to a different city?
- Do I have reliable transportation to get to and from a job?
- How many miles am I willing to commute each way?
- Do I need full-time or part-time work?
- Will I need to find child care?
- Do I have backup child care for summers, when a child is sick from school, and so on?

Most people will not be able to compromise on some of these items. Though a new job may sound enticing, if it requires relocation or a long commute, it might not be a good match for your needs. Though child care is tax deductible, a new graduate might not be able to afford the weekly costs associated with child care. Determine your needs and make a list. Use this list to help you determine the best jobs for which you should apply.

Where to Look for a Job

Externship sites often can provide leading sources for jobs after graduation. Though not all externship sites have the availability to offer a student a position upon graduation, it is possible that the office manager or physician at the externship site might be aware of another office that is looking to hire. A professional and confident student should be able to ask the office managers or physicians if they are able to recommend a specific medical office or facility that may be hiring. This is also a good time to ask if they would be willing to serve as a professional reference related to your externship experience.

Local newspapers are another great source for medical assistant positions. *Help wanted* ads are often found within the Classified section of a newspaper. Furthermore, medical assistant jobs are most often placed in the medical/healthcare sections of the classified ads. Often, the newspaper will also post help wanted ads on its Web site. While perusing classified ads, keep a close eye on the job location and hours of work.

The Internet is a tremendous resource during a job search. Popular search engines such as Monster, CareerBuilder, and Simply Hired offer great starting points for medical assistant jobs. Additionally, it is helpful to check out Web sites of local hospitals, medical offices, and other medical facilities within your community. If you don't know the exact Web site of a company, typing in the business name and location into an Internet search engine will often help find the company's main Web site.

Local staffing agencies are another option during the job search. A **staffing agency** is a third party that has been hired by an employer to find employees to fill certain positions. Sometimes these positions are **temporary jobs**, sometimes referred to as temp jobs, meaning they are only for a specific amount of time, such as three to six months. Temporary jobs may also be termed **temp-to-hire**, meaning the position has the possibility of turning into a permanent position.

Finally, many schools offer career assistance services. These services have been specifically created to help new graduates find gainful employment within their field. School representatives form professional relationships with companies and facilities within the area. The reputation of the school and the graduates plays a major factor in a company's willingness to work with a school. Medical offices that work directly with a school will contact the director of career services when a position needs to be filled. After all information has been obtained from the employer, the career services representative will often speak with department heads and instructors to help find suitable candidates to apply for the position. Again, this is an instance where displaying competence and professionalism as a student will help your employability chances after graduation.

Networking

Networking is a tool used by professionals to engage with other like-minded individuals within their field of expertise to create business contacts for the purpose of working together in joint business ventures. The key to networking is getting to know people within your field and making purposeful contacts with them. For the medical assistant, this might be accomplished by joining local chapters of professional organizations such as the American Association of Medical Assistants, American Medical Technologists, or the American Academy of Professional Coders. Community involvement and volunteering in the areas of community healthcare, hospitals, and clinics provide other avenues for networking as a medical assistant. When someone makes a new contact, it is important to make a positive first impression. This can be done by making direct eye contact, presenting a firm handshake, and smiling while making introductions. While introductions are being made, tell the fellow person your name, your credentials, and where you work. It is helpful to have personal business cards for the purpose of networking. Personal business cards do not list your current employer, but rather include your personal contact information such as your name, personal email address, personal telephone number, and personal Web site.

Confidence versus Arrogance

It is important that new graduates looking to secure a position in the field of medical assisting understand the difference between confidence with arrogance. **Confidence** is positively portraying personal skills and qualities with dignity while maintaining an air of self-worth and grace. On the other hand, **arrogance** is a lofty attitude characterized by bragging and an unnecessary sense of entitlement.

Career Tips

Be prepared!—When scouring the newspaper, online job boards, and local career centers for a job in your field, be prepared to match your job desires and skills with those that are available for hire. Take the time to answer some simple questions and set **parameters**, or boundaries, regarding your availability and skill set. Starting off in the field, you will not be qualified for jobs that require experienced medical assistants. However, if you truly believe the job to be a good personal fit for your skill set and if you have a desire and gumption to apply as a motivated new graduate, eager to learn, you may be surprised that you still can land a job! The exercise at the end of this chapter will help you get on your way to establishing your skills and career desires.

It is important to highlight skills and achievements as a new graduate. The confusion arises in how this information is given to a prospective new employer. Often times, when applicants give off a sense of arrogance, they will almost immediately be eliminated from the job pool due to the fact that many people who are thought of as arrogant are also perceived as difficult to work with and not considered as team players. An example of confidence versus arrogance was cited in Chapter 1; however, because this is such an important concept, another example has been presented here (see Box 2-1).

BOX 2-1 Confidence versus Arrogance in Action

Marcus had a wonderful experience during his medical assisting externship. Unfortunately, the site was unable to offer him a position after Marcus's graduation. The office manager of the externship site wrote Marcus a very thoughtful letter of recommendation and encouraged Marcus by saying she would act as a professional reference during his job hunt. Two weeks after graduation, Marcus was able to get an interview at an endocrinology office that has a wonderful reputation in the community for not only treating their patients with care but also supporting and encouraging their employees. During his interview Marcus was asked to describe his experience during his externship.

Marcus's confident response: "I had a wonderful experience at my externship site. I was able to learn a lot from both the doctors and staff. I found that I have strong clinical skills and I enjoy working with patients of all ages. I have a letter of recommendation from the office manager of my externship site that I would be happy to share with you."

Marcus's arrogant response: "I was really great during my externship. It seemed like I knew everything that they were trying to teach me. I was one of the best members of the clinical team, even better than their current staff members. The office manager was so impressed by my skills that she wrote me a letter of recommendation."

Mentoring

After gaining employment, it is important and incredibly beneficial to have a mentor in your new office. In addition to on-the-job training, a **mentor** will provide advice and assistance in navigating the politics of the medical office. One of the hardest jobs of a mentor is to provide constructive criticism. Everyone has areas in which they need to improve. It is the job of the mentor to provide recommendations and suggestions on ways to improve personal, professional, or competency-related behaviors.

Training in the Office

A mentor will be the medical assistant's prime source of information and training in the office. It is reasonable to expect a thirty- to sixty-day training period. Often, many offices require demonstrated competence in a specific skill set before a new hire is allowed to work completely on his or her own. See ■ Figure 2-1 for an example of a competency checklist. When observing the responsibilities and duties performed during the job, the newly hired medical assistant will learn the policies and procedures for specific tasks that may vary from office to office.

During the observation and training period, any questions regarding policies, procedures, and protocols should be asked. Many new hires are intimidated to ask questions because they feel it makes them look unintelligent or unprepared. In actuality, the new hire who asks questions will gain more respect in the office because his or her teammates will recognize that the medical assistant is not willing to risk wasted time or compromise patient care over a sensitive ego.

The job of the mentor is not complete once the medical assistant has mastered the necessary list of required competencies. A true mentor will continue to be a source of guidance and help throughout the medical assistant's career.

Displaying Competence

Competence is having the ability or aptitude to perform a skill. After you have finished training and demonstrating your abilities, it is important to continue to display competence when working on your own. Not only is it important to show the physician, office manager, or fellow coworkers your abilities, it is also important for patients to see your competence.

Many patients suffer from white-coat syndrome. This is characterized by anxiety and uneasiness when around doctors and medical staff. In some patients, white-coat syndrome manifests through increased blood pressure and anxiety. Other patients simply avoid doctors all together. A medical assistant who is able to effectively display competence when working with patients can help decrease the level of anxiety a patient may feel simply by being at the doctor's office. ■ Table 2-1 describes ways a medical assistant can display competence with patients.

Pearson Medical Group
New Hire Competency CheckList

Name: Malinda Peterson, RMA
Date of Hire: 11/12/2012
Training with: Lilly Aquilla, CMA(AAMA)

Skill	Observed #1	Observed #2	Practice #1	Practice #2	Practice #11
Schedule a New Patient	11/14/2012 Lilly A., CMA(AAMA)	11/14/2012 Lilly A., CMA(AAMA)	11/16/2012 Lilly A., CMA(AAMA)	11/19/2012 Lilly A., CMA(AAMA)	
Schedule an Existing Patient	11/14/2012 Lilly A., CMA(AAMA)	11/14/2012 Lilly A., CMA(AAMA)	11/16/2012 Lilly A., CMA(AAMA)	11/16/2012 Lilly A., CMA(AAMA)	11/16/2012 Lilly A., CMA(AAMA)
Complete the check-out process for a patient, including rescheduling an appointment.	11/22/2012 Lilly A., CMA(AAMA)	11/22/2012 Lilly A., CMA(AAMA)			
Create a New Patient Chart	11/14/2012 Lilly A., CMA(AAMA)	11/14/2012 Lilly A., CMA(AAMA)	11/16/2012 Lilly A., CMA(AAMA)	11/19/2012 Lilly A., CMA(AAMA)	
Obtain Vitals	11/19/2012 Lilly A., CMA(AAMA)				
Obtain a CC	11/19/2012 Lilly A., CMA(AAMA)				
Obtain blood sample via vacutainer					
Obtain blood sample via butterfly method					
Perform a visual acuity test					

■ FIGURE 2-1

Example of a new hire competency checklist.

■ TABLE 2-1 **Displaying Competence with Patients**

Always make eye contact.	Making eye contact demonstrates self-confidence, which is important in displaying competence. Also, it shows respect for your patients.
Be truthful about errors.	If a mistake has been made, be truthful with the patient. Many patients will be understanding and respect the fact that you did not hide your mistakes.
If you do not know, ask!	Oftentimes a patient will ask a medical assistant questions regarding his or her health status. It is important not to pretend to know information or make up information that you believe to be correct. The best thing to do when a patient asks a question that you are unable to answer is to tell the patient that you do not know and you will ask the doctor on the patient's behalf.

END OF CHAPTER REVIEW

LEARNING OBJECTIVE REVIEW

Complete each learning objective to the best of your ability.

1. Explain the importance of understanding a personal skill set.

_____

_____

_____

_____

_____

2. Identify why it is important to recognize personal limitations when applying for a job.

_____

_____

_____

_____

_____

3. List and describe four of the five resources that are helpful when beginning a job search.

_____

_____

_____

_____

_____

4. Describe the difference between confidence and arrogance.

_____

_____

_____

_____

_____

5. Explain the duties of a mentor.

_____

_____

_____

_____

_____

KEY TERMS

Use each of the following key terms in a sentence that demonstrates your understanding of the word.

1. arrogance:_____

_____

2. competence:_____

_____

3. confidence:_____

_____

4. mentor:_____

_____

5. networking:_____

_____

6. parameters:_____

_____

7. role model:_____

_____

8. skill set:_____

_____

9. staffing agency:_____

_____

10. temporary job:_____

_____

11. temp-to-hire:_____

_____

CRITICAL THINKING

Reread the workplace scenario at the beginning of the chapter and answer the following questions.

1. What type of skill set should Sue Ellen have in order to be an effective employee should she be offered the position after her interview?

_____

_____

_____

_____

2. Sue Ellen lives alone in her apartment and does not have health insurance benefits. Should this be of concern when she considers accepting the position at the pediatric office?

_____

_____

_____

_____

3. Sue Ellen graduated at the top of her class from Pearson Community College. She received various awards and accolades for both her academic achievements and her community involvement. How should Sue Ellen approach this during her interview?

_____

_____

_____

DO IT YOURSELF!

Complete the modules below to demonstrate your understanding of the chapter.

Module A

Complete the following questioners regarding your personal skill set and employment goals. What type of jobs will you be most suited for in the medical office?

A-1. Skill Set Questionnaire

Take the time to consider your answers to these questions. The answers that you give will help steer you toward the area of medical assisting that is best for you.

1. Which do you prefer?
   a. Clinical medical assisting (continue to question #2 and skip #3)
   b. Administrative medical assisting (continue to question #3 and skip #2)
   c. I like both (complete both questions #2 and #3)

2. Clinical medical assisting: Check each of the following skills you enjoy performing:
   ☐ Vital signs (TPR-BP)
   ☐ Examination assistance (assisting during PAP exams, physical exams, sigmoidoscopies, etc.)
   ☐ Injections (adult)
   ☐ Injections (pediatric)
   ☐ Phlebotomy (adult)
   ☐ Phlebotomy (pediatric)
   ☐ Special ordered tests or treatments (EKGs, spirometry, nebulizer treatments, etc.)
   ☐ Lab tests (random blood glucose, urinalysis, ESR, etc.)

3. Administrative medical assisting: Check each of the following skills you enjoy performing:
   ☐ Answering phones
   ☐ Returning messages for the doctor
   ☐ Scheduling office appointments
   ☐ Scheduling outpatient examinations and tests
   ☐ Performing checkout duties (collecting co-pays, posting payments, scheduling follow-up appointments, etc.)
   ☐ Medical billing and coding
   ☐ Medical transcription
   ☐ Working with medical insurance companies (obtaining precertifications, following up on medical claims, etc.)
   ☐ Records management (making new charts, filing charts, handling requests for medical records, etc.)

4. Summarize your ideal job responsibilities:

_____

_____

_____

5. Are you competent in your ideal job responsibilities?

_____

_____

_____

A-2. Employment Worksheet

The following questions will help you identify your employment needs. Consider your current living situation and what your situation will be on graduation. The answers to these questions will help you identify the ideal jobs you should apply for.

1. Do you need full-time or part-time work? _____

2. Do you need health insurance benefits? _____ *(If yes, keep in mind that most companies offer health insurance only to full-time employees.)*

3. What days are you available to work?
   - ☐ Monday
   - ☐ Tuesday
   - ☐ Wednesday
   - ☐ Thursday
   - ☐ Friday
   - ☐ Saturday
   - ☐ Sunday

4. Are you available to work
   - ☐ mornings?
   - ☐ afternoons?
   - ☐ evenings?

5. Do you drive? _____

6. Do you have reliable transportation? _____

7. Identify an acceptable commute time: _____

8. Do you need to arrange child care? _____

9. Will you have a plan in place for backup child care? _____

10. Would you like to work in a
    ☐ doctor's office?
    ☐ hospital?
    ☐ laboratory?

11. Do you have a preference to certain fields of healthcare?
    ☐ Pediatrics
    ☐ Family medicine
    ☐ Obstetrics/gynecology
    ☐ Gastrointestinal
    ☐ Ophthalmology
    ☐ Pulmonary medicine
    ☐ Other:_____

12. Do you wish to continue your education? If yes, what would you like to do? _____
    _____

    Based on your answers to questions 1 to 12, summarize your ideal employment situation. Where will it be located, will it be a specialty office, how many hours will you be working and on which days? Use this information to help guide you as you are looking for jobs in the field of medical assisting.

    _____

    _____

    _____

    _____

Module B

Create a help wanted ad that would be ideal for your skill set and employment goals. Be sure to list all the information that would be provided in a real help wanted advertisement.

_____

_____

_____

_____

_____

_____

_____

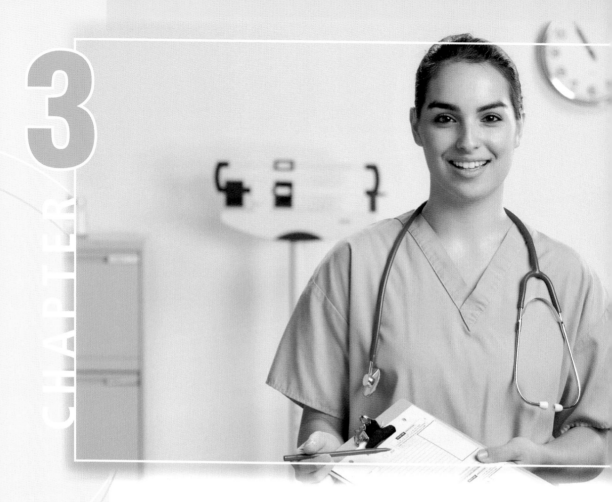

Professionalism among Coworkers

LEARNING OBJECTIVES

- Explain the significance of a chain of command within an office environment.
- Describe elements of appropriate workplace conversations.
- Describe how to appropriately address physicians.
- Discuss issues involved with communicating patient information.
- List examples of how to handle various difficult situations in the workplace.
- Discuss sexual harassment in the workplace.

Workplace Scenario

Marla is a medical assistant working for a pediatric office. She has just finished administering two immunizations to a 12-month-old, baby girl. Her coworker and fellow medical assistant, Alicia, helped to hold the baby to prevent injury while Marla administered the immunizations. Later in the day, Marla overhears Alicia say the following to a fellow coworker: "You should have seen Marla giving that baby those shots; she had no idea what she was doing. I feel sorry for that kid. If I were the mother, I'd never bring my child back to this office."

Introduction

When working in the medical office, you may find that some of the most difficult situations that you encounter involve your coworkers. This chapter will prepare you to interact both appropriately and professionally with your coworkers as well as handle various situations that may arise in the workplace.

Office Structure

Chains of command may vary among medical offices. Miscommunication may occur due to lack of communication or not understanding a **chain of command**. The chain of command refers to the ranking of authority within the office. ■ Figure 3-1 illustrates an example of a typical chain of command in a medical office. Chains of command may vary from office to office. It is important to find out not only the chain of command in the office where you work but also where you perform your **practicum**, or externship.

An integral part to professionalism among coworkers involves the ability to not only understand but also accept the role of your **supervisor**. When a person has accepted the role of

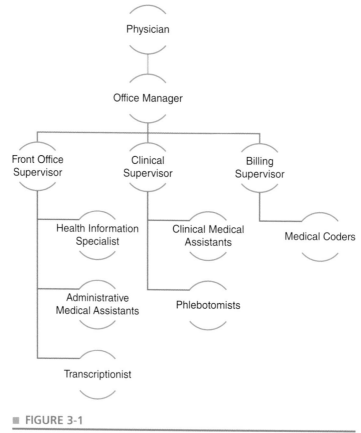

■ FIGURE 3-1

An example of a chain of command in a typical medical office.

supervisor, he or she has agreed to take on additional responsibilities within the office. General responsibilities of a supervisor include the following:

- Implementing policies and procedures
- Establishing a work schedule, which includes reviewing staffing needs and making adjustments as necessary
- New employee training
- Handling immediate patient concerns
- Ensuring that staff members work safely, cohesively, and productively

It is important to direct any concerns or problems that you have to your immediate supervisor. If a particular situation is beyond the control of your immediate supervisor, he or she will likely report the issue to his or her immediate supervisor, and so on up the chain of command until the issue has been resolved. It is considered unprofessional to break the chain of command within the office setting. If issues occur with coworkers during the practicum or externship experience, it is necessary to continue to follow the chain of command that is established in the office. Should students experience problematic situations at an externship site, they should report them to their academic advisor or externship coordinator. The ability to be forthcoming about such situations is another component of professionalism on behalf of the student.

Interacting with Coworkers

Two very important items to remember while working in the medical office are that (1) the medical office is a place for work, not for socializing with your closest friends, and (2) you can pick your friends, but not your coworkers. There are many benefits to getting along well with those whom you work with. Respecting your coworkers is essential in the office setting. When you show respect for your coworkers, they will likely, in turn, show respect for you. This helps build a strong foundation for teamwork. ■ Table 3-1 illustrates six ways you can show respect

■ TABLE 3-1 **Six Ways to Show Respect to Your Coworkers**

Technique	Technique in Action
1. Maintain their confidence.	If a coworker shares a personal matter or concern with you, keep it private.
2. Respect their personal space.	Everyone needs to have his or her own personal space; allow coworkers theirs. Try not to infringe on their personal work space or areas where they store their personal belongings.
3. Be helpful and courteous.	Offer help when you see a coworker struggling and always say "thank you" when someone helps you. A little bit of courtesy can go a long way.
4. Keep your language clean.	Do not curse or use foul language, ever. Many people do not appreciate it, in any setting.
5. Be aware of their feelings.	Sarcasm, jokes, and making fun can truly hurt people even if it is spoken in jest. Do not take a person's feelings for granted by assuming he or she will think a joke is funny. Take the higher ground and show true respect by not making other people the butt of jokes.
6. Take responsibility.	Everyone will make mistakes. It is an inevitable component of being human. When you make a mistake, own up to it. Accept the blame and consequences with dignity, rather than trying to pass the blame onto someone else.

for your coworkers. Oftentimes it is easier to resolve conflicts, and a "teamwork" atmosphere may be more apparent.

Coworkers have many opportunities to interact and converse. Often, however, the line may be crossed regarding appropriate interaction. To ensure that a conversation is appropriate consider the following questions:

- Can this conversation be discussed with the entire medical office?
- Could anyone be offended by what is being said?
- Would this conversation be given a "PG" rating?
- Would I feel comfortable if this conversation were published in a local newspaper available for everyone to read?

If you are able to answer "yes" to all of the above questions, then the conversation would most likely be considered permissible to have with your coworkers and in the presence of others. Personal conversations between coworkers pertaining to private matters should *never* be discussed in main office areas. This includes the reception area, the front office, the back office, hallways, and examination rooms. Personal conversations shared with coworkers should remain confidential and not be repeated without permission. The only exception to this would be if the information shared by a coworker could affect the person's ability to perform his or her job or damage the integrity of the medical practice. However, such assumptions should be made only after thoughtful consideration. Careful thought must be given regarding how to handle the situation by causing the least amount of damage. A situational example is found in the End of the Chapter Review, Apply Your Knowledge #5.

Gossip

Along with inappropriate conversations, **gossip** has no place in the medical office. Gossip is needless chatter that can lead to rumors, especially regarding someone's personal life. It can be very difficult to avoid; however, the professional medical assistant should take a higher ground and refuse to participate or listen to gossip that may circulate in the workplace. Gossip can not only be damaging to a person's character, but it can also deteriorate the rapport among coworkers.

Students working at an externship site should never be involved with office gossip. Not only will this behavior damage their professional image, but it will likely prevent them from being offered a position within the office should one become available as office managers and supervisors are aware of those in the office who engage in gossip. Additionally, the office manager may contact the student's school with concerns regarding the student's interoffice interactions, and it could affect the student's final externship grade.

Addressing Physicians

While employed as a medical assistant, physicians within the office should be viewed not only as authority figures but also as coworkers with whom you must interact. As a rule of thumb, it is never fitting that you address a physician by his or her first name. Addressing a physician by saying "Doctor" before his or her last name is considered professional as well as respectful: for example, "Good morning, Doctor LaFaro." In some cases, a physician may ask to be called by his or her first name, in which case an appropriate greeting may be "Good morning, Doctor Joe."

Communicating Patient Information

Many times, you will find it necessary to discuss **confidential** patient information with your coworkers. It is illegal to breach patient confidentiality as outlined by the **Health Insurance Portability and Accountability Act (HIPAA)**, which was passed in August of 1996. Over the past few years, patients have become more and more familiar with the rules and laws associated with HIPAA, as well as their rights. If a patient feels as though confidentiality pertaining to his or her healthcare has been breached, he or she has the opportunity to file a complaint with the **Office for Civil Rights (OCR)**, a division of the **U.S. Department of Health and Human Services**. ■ Figure 3-2 shows the Health Information Privacy Complaint Form that was created by the Office of Civil Rights. Those who breach patient confidentiality risk not only losing their jobs but also possible **litigation**.

When communicating confidential patient information adhere to the following principles:

- Remember that just because someone works in a medical office does not allow him or her access to all patient medical files.
- A healthcare professional should have access to patient files only when he or she is directly involved in the patient's care.
- Communicate patient information only with those who need to have direct contact with the patient in order to provide healthcare.
- Share *only* the information that is needed.
- Do not discuss confidential patient information within hearing range of anyone not associated with the patient's care.
- If it is necessary to fax patient information to healthcare providers, always use a HIPAA **compliant** fax cover sheet.

Interacting with a Difficult Coworker

As mentioned earlier in the chapter, there are two crucial items to remember when working in a medical office. The second crucial item to remember is that *you can pick your friends, but not your coworkers*. It is virtually inevitable that at some point in your life you will encounter a difficult coworker. Though this can be difficult to deal with, having a positive and professional approach to the situation can be an invaluable asset.

Handling a Problematic Situation

When encountered with a difficult situation at work, the manner in which you handle both the issue and yourself will affect the outcome. It is always best to speak directly with the person who is problematic and not others. ■ Table 3-2 provides five steps for resolving conflict with a co-worker. As we discussed earlier, gossip has detrimental effects on a workplace. Always approach the "offender" in a calm manner. If you are unable to speak in a calm manner immediately, postpone the discussion until you have had a chance to relax and collect your thoughts. If you

DEPARTMENT OF HEALTH AND HUMAN SERVICES
OFFICE FOR CIVIL RIGHTS (OCR)

Form Approved: OMB No. 0990-0269.
SeeOMBStatementonReverse.

HEALTH INFORMATION PRIVACY COMPLAINT

YOUR FIRST NAME

YOUR LAST NAME

HOME PHONE (Please include area code)

WORK PHONE (Please include area code)

STREET ADDRESS

CITY

STATE

ZIP

E-MAIL ADDRESS (If available)

Are you filing this complaint for someone else? ☐ Yes   ☐ No
If Yes, whose health information privacy rights do you believe were violated?

FIRST NAME

LAST NAME

Who (or what agency or organization, e.g., provider, health plan) do you believe violated your (or someone else's) health information privacy rights or committed another violation of the Privacy Rule?
PERSON / AGENCY / ORGANIZATION

STREET ADDRESS

CITY

STATE

ZIP

PHONE (Please include area code)

When do you believe that the violation of health information privacy rights occurred?
LIST DATE(S)

Describe briefly what happened. How and why do you believe your (or someone else's) health information privacy rights were violated, or the privacy rule otherwise was violated? Please be as specific as possible. (Attach additional pages as needed)

Please sign and date this complaint. You do not need to sign if submitting this form by email because submission by email represents your signature.
SIGNATURE

DATE

The remaining information on this form is optional. Failure to answer these voluntary questions will not affect OCR's decision to process your complaint.

Do you need special accommodations for OCR to communicate with you about this complaint? (Check all that apply)

☐ Braille   ☐ Large Print   ☐ Cassette tape   ☐ Computer diskette   ☐ Electronic mail   ☐ TDD

☐ Sign language interpreter (specify language): _____

☐ Foreign language interpreter (specify language): _____   ☐ Other: _____

If we cannot reach you directly, is there someone we can contact to help us reach you?

FIRST NAME	LAST NAME
HOME PHONE (Please include area code)	WORK PHONE (Please include area code)
STREET ADDRESS	CITY
STATE ZIP	E-MAIL ADDRESS (If available)

Have you filed your complaint anywhere else? If so, please provide the following. (Attach additional pages as needed)
PERSON / AGENCY / ORGANIZATION / COURT NAME(S)

DATE(S) FILED	CASE NUMBER(S) (If known)

To help us better serve the public, please provide the following information for the person you believe had their health information privacy rights violated (you or the person on whose behalf you are filing).

ETHNICITY (select one)   RACE (select one or more)

☐ Hispanic or Latino   ☐ American Indian or Alaska Native   ☐ Asian   ☐ Native Hawaiian or Other Pacific Islander

☐ Not Hispanic or Latino   ☐ Black or African American   ☐ White   ☐ Other (specify): _____

PRIMARY LANGUAGE SPOKEN (if other than English) _____

How did you learn about the Office for Civil Rights?

☐ HHS Website / Internet Search   ☐ Family / Friend/Associate   ☐ Religious/Community Org   ☐ Lawyer / Legal Org   ☐ Phone Directory   ☐ Employer

☐ Fed/State / Local Gov   ☐ Healthcare Provider / Health Plan   ☐ Conference / OCR Brochure   ☐ Other (specify): _____

To mail a complaint, please type or print, and return completed complaint to the OCR Regional Address based on the region where the alleged discrimination took place. If you need assistance completing this form, contact the appropriate region listed below.

Region I - CT, ME, MA, NH, RI, VT Office for Civil Rights, DHHS JFK Federal Building - Room 1875 Boston, MA 02203 (617) 565-1340; (617) 565-1343 (TDD) (617) 565-3809 FAX	**Region V - IL, IN, MI, MN, OH, WI** Office for Civil Rights, DHHS 233 N. Michigan Ave. - Suite 240 Chicago, IL 60601 (312) 886-2359; (312) 353-5693 (TDD) (312) 886-1807 FAX	**Region IX - AZ, CA, HI, NV, AS, GU,** **The U.S. Affiliated Pacific Island Jurisdictions** Office for Civil Rights, DHHS 90 7th Street, Suite 4-100 San Francisco, CA 94103 (415) 437-8310; (415) 437-8311 (TDD) (415) 437-8329 FAX
Region II - NJ, NY, PR, VI Office for Civil Rights, DHHS 26 Federal Plaza - Suite 3313 New York, NY 10278 (212) 264-3313; (212) 264-2355 (TDD) (212) 264-3039 FAX	**Region VI - AR, LA, NM, OK, TX** Office for Civil Rights, DHHS 1301 Young Street - Suite 1169 Dallas, TX 75202 (214) 767-4056; (214) 767-8940 (TDD) (214) 767-0432 FAX	
Region III - DE, DC, MD, PA, VA, WV Office for Civil Rights, DHHS 150 S. Independence Mall West - Suite 372 Philadelphia, PA 19106-3499 (215) 861-4441; (215) 861-4440 (TDD) (215) 861-4431 FAX	**Region VII - IA, KS, MO, NE** Office for Civil Rights, DHHS 601 East 12th Street - Room 248 Kansas City, MO 64106 (816) 426-7277; (816) 426-7065 (TDD) (816) 426-3686 FAX	
Region IV - AL, FL, GA, KY, MS, NC, SC, TN Office for Civil Rights, DHHS 61 Forsyth Street, SW. - Suite 3B70 Atlanta, GA 30303-8909 (404) 562-7886; (404) 331-2867 (TDD) (404) 562-7881 FAX	**Region VIII - CO, MT, ND, SD, UT, WY** Office for Civil Rights, DHHS 1961 Stout Street - Room 1426 Denver, CO 80294 (303) 844-2024; (303) 844-3439 (TDD) (303) 844-2025 FAX	**Region X - AK, ID, OR, WA** Office for Civil Rights, DHHS 2201 Sixth Avenue - Mail Stop RX-11 Seattle, WA 98121 (206) 615-2290; (206) 615-2296 (TDD) (206) 615-2297 FAX

Burden Statement

Public reporting burden for the collection of information on this complaint form is estimated to average 45 minutes per response, including the time for reviewing instructions, gathering the data needed and entering and reviewing the information on the completed complaint form. An agency may not conduct or sponsor, and a person is not required to respond to, a collection of information unless it displays a valid control number. Send comments regarding this burden estimate or any other aspect of this collection of information, including suggestions for reducing this burden, to: HHS/OS Reports Clearance Officer, Office of Information Resources Management, 200 Independence Ave. S.W., Room 531H, Washington, D.C. 20201.

HHS-700 (6/08) (BACK)

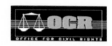

COMPLAINANT CONSENT FORM

The Department of Health and Human Services' (HHS) Office for Civil Rights (OCR) has the authority to collect and receive material and information about you, including personnel and medical records, which are relevant to its investigation of your complaint.

To investigate your complaint, OCR may need to reveal your identity or identifying information about you to persons at the entity or agency under investigation or to other persons, agencies, or entities.

The Privacy Act of 1974 protects certain federal records that contain personally identifiable information about you and, with your consent, allows OCR to use your name or other personal information, if necessary, to investigate your complaint.

Consent is voluntary, and it is not always needed in order to investigate your complaint; however, failure to give consent is likely to impede the investigation of your complaint and may result in the closure of your case.

Additionally, OCR may disclose information, including medical records and other personal information, which it has gathered during the course of its investigation in order to comply with a request under the Freedom of Information Act (FOIA) and may refer your complaint to another appropriate agency.

Under FOIA, OCR may be required to release information regarding the investigation of your complaint; however, we will make every effort, as permitted by law, to protect information that identifies individuals or that, if released, could constitute a clearly unwarranted invasion of personal privacy.

Please read and review the documents entitled, *Protecting Personal Information in Complaint Investigations* and *Notice to Complainants and Other Individuals Asked to Supply Information to the Office for Civil Rights* for further information regarding how OCR may obtain, use, and disclose your information while investigating your complaint.

In order to expedite the investigation of your complaint if it is accepted by OCR, please read, sign, and return one copy of this consent form to OCR with your complaint. Please make one copy for your records.

- As a complainant, I understand that in the course of the investigation of my complaint it may become necessary for OCR to reveal my identity or identifying information about me to persons at the entity or agency under investigation or to other persons, agencies, or entities.

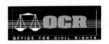

- I am also aware of the obligations of OCR to honor requests under the Freedom of Information Act (FOIA). I understand that it may be necessary for OCR to disclose information, including personally identifying information, which it has gathered as part of its investigation of my complaint.

- In addition, I understand that as a complainant I am covered by the Department of Health and Human Services' (HHS) regulations which protect any individual from being intimidated, threatened, coerced, retaliated against, or discriminated against because he/she has made a complaint, testified, assisted, or participated in any manner in any mediation, investigation, hearing, proceeding, or other part of HHS' investigation, conciliation, or enforcement process.

After reading the above information, please check ONLY ONE of the following boxes:

☐ **CONSENT**: I have read, understand, and agree to the above and give permission to OCR to reveal my identity or identifying information about me in my case file to persons at the entity or agency under investigation or to other relevant persons, agencies, or entities during any part of HHS' investigation, conciliation, or enforcement process.

☐ **CONSENT DENIED**: I have read and I understand the above and do not give permission to OCR to reveal my identity or identifying information about me. I understand that this denial of consent is likely to impede the investigation of my complaint and may result in closure of the investigation.

Signature: _____ Date: _____

*Please sign and date this complaint. You do not need to sign if submitting this form by email because submission by email represents your signature.

Name (Please type or print): _____

Address: _____

Telephone Number: _____

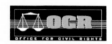

NOTICE TO COMPLAINANTS AND OTHER
INDIVIDUALS ASKED TO SUPPLY INFORMATION
TO THE OFFICE FOR CIVIL RIGHTS

Privacy Act

The Privacy Act of 1974 (5 U.S.C. §552a) requires OCR to notify individuals whom it asks to supply information that:

— OCR is authorized to solicit information under:
(i) Federal laws barring discrimination by recipients of Federal financial assistance on grounds of race, color, national origin, disability, age, sex, religion under programs and activities receiving Federal financial assistance from the U.S. Department of Health and Human Services (HHS), including, but not limited to, Title VI of the Civil Rights Act of 1964 (42 U.S.C. §2000d et seq.), Section 504 of the Rehabilitation Act of 1973 (29 U.S.C. §794), the Age Discrimination Act of 1975 (42 U.S.C. §6101 et seq.), Title IX of the Education Amendments of 1972 (20 U.S.C. §1681 et seq.), and Sections 794 and 855 of the Public Health Service Act (42 U.S.C. §§295m and 296g);
(ii) Titles VI and XVI of the Public Health Service Act (42 U.S.C. §§291 et seq. and 300s et seq.) and 42 C.F.R. Part 124, Subpart G (Community Service obligations of Hill-Burton facilities);
(iii) 45 C.F.R. Part 85, as it implements Section 504 of the Rehabilitation Act in programs conducted by HHS; and
(iv) Title II of the Americans with Disabilities Act (42 U.S.C. §12131 et seq.) and Department of Justice regulations at 28 C.F.R. Part 35, which give HHS "designated agency" authority to investigate and resolve disability discrimination complaints against certain public entities, defined as health and service agencies of state and local governments, regardless of whether they receive federal financial assistance.
(v) The Standards for the Privacy of Individually Identifiable Health Information (The Privacy Rule) at 45 C.F.R. Part 160 and Subparts A and E of Part 164, which enforce the Health Insurance Portability and Accountability Act of 1996 (HIPAA) (42 U.S.C. §1320d-2).

OCR will request information for the purpose of determining and securing compliance with the Federal laws listed above. Disclosure of this requested information to OCR by individuals who are not recipients of federal financial assistance is voluntary; however, even individuals who voluntarily disclose information are subject to prosecution and penalties under 18 U.S.C. § 1001 for making false statements.

Additionally, although disclosure is voluntary for individuals who are not recipients of federal financial assistance, failure to provide OCR with requested information may preclude OCR from making a compliance determination or enforcing the laws above.

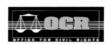

OCR has the authority to disclose personal information collected during an investigation without the individual's consent for the following routine uses:

(i) to make disclosures to OCR contractors who are required to maintain Privacy Act safeguards with respect to such records;
(ii) for disclosure to a congressional office from the record of an individual in response to an inquiry made at the request of the individual;
(iii) to make disclosures to the Department of Justice to permit effective defense of litigation; and
(iv) to make disclosures to the appropriate agency in the event that records maintained by OCR to carry out its functions indicate a violation or potential violation of law.

Under 5 U.S.C. §552a(k)(2) and the HHS Privacy Act regulations at 45 C.F.R. §5b.11 OCR complaint records have been exempted as investigatory material compiled for law enforcement purposes from certain Privacy Act access, amendment, correction and notification requirements.

Freedom of Information Act
A complainant, the recipient or any member of the public may request release of OCR records under the Freedom of Information Act (5 U.S.C. §552) (FOIA) and HHS regulations at 45 C.F.R. Part 5.

Fraud and False Statements
Federal law, at 18 U.S.C. §1001, authorizes prosecution and penalties of fine or imprisonment for conviction of "whoever, in any matter within the jurisdiction of any department or agency of the United States knowingly and willfully falsifies, conceals or covers up by any trick, scheme, or device a material fact, or makes any false, fictitious or fraudulent statements or representations or makes or uses any false writing or document knowing the same to contain any false, fictitious, or fraudulent statement or entry".

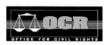

PROTECTING PERSONAL INFORMATION IN COMPLAINT INVESTIGATIONS

To investigate your complaint, the Department of Health and Human Services' (HHS) Office for Civil Rights (OCR) will collect information from different sources. Depending on the type of complaint, we may need to get copies of your medical records, or other information that is personal to you. This Fact Sheet explains how OCR protects your personal information that is part of your case file.

HOW DOES OCR PROTECT MY PERSONAL INFORMATION?

OCR is required by law to protect your personal information. The Privacy Act of 1974 protects Federal records about an individual containing personally identifiable information, including, but not limited to, the individual's medical history, education, financial transactions, and criminal or employment history that contains an individual's name or other identifying information.

Because of the Privacy Act, OCR will use your name or other personal information with a signed consent and only when it is necessary to complete the investigation of your complaint or to enforce civil rights laws or when it is otherwise permitted by law.

Consent is voluntary, and it is not always needed in order to investigate your complaint; however, failure to give consent is likely to impede the investigation of your complaint and may result in the closure of your case.

CAN I SEE MY OCR FILE?

Under the Freedom of Information Act (FOIA), you can request a copy of your case file once your case has been closed; however, OCR can withhold information from you in order to protect the identities of witnesses and other sources of information.

CAN OCR GIVE MY FILE TO ANY ONE ELSE?

If a complaint indicates a violation or a potential violation of law, OCR can refer the complaint to another appropriate agency without your permission.

If you file a complaint with OCR, and we decide we cannot help you, we may refer your complaint to another agency such as the Department of Justice.

CAN ANYONE ELSE SEE THE INFORMATION IN MY FILE?

Access to OCR's files and records is controlled by the Freedom of Information Act (FOIA). Under FOIA, OCR may be required to release information about this case upon public request. In the event that OCR receives such a request, we will make every effort,

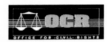

as permitted by law, to protect information that identifies individuals, or that, if released, could constitute a clearly unwarranted invasion of personal privacy.

If OCR receives protected health information about you in connection with a HIPAA Privacy Rule investigation or compliance review, we will only share this information with individuals outside of HHS if necessary for our compliance efforts or if we are required to do so by another law.

DOES IT COST ANYTHING FOR ME (OR SOMEONE ELSE) TO OBTAIN A COPY OF MY FILE?

In most cases, the first two hours spent searching for document(s) you request under the Freedom of Information Act and the first 100 pages are free. Additional search time or copying time may result in a cost for which you will be responsible. If you wish to limit the search time and number of pages to a maximum of two hours and 100 pages; please specify this in your request. You may also set a specific cost limit, for example, cost not to exceed $100.00.

If you have any questions about this fact sheet, please contact OCR
http://www.hhs.gov/ocr/contact.html

OR

Contact your OCR Regional Office
(see Regional Office contact information on page 2 of the Complaint Form)

■ FIGURE 3-2

The Health Information Privacy Complaint Form created by the Office of Civil Rights.

Source: http://www.hhs.gov/ocr/privacy/hipaa/complaints/hipcomplaintpackage.pdf

---

■ TABLE 3-2 **Five Steps to Resolving Conflicts with Coworkers**

1. Identify the problem. Keep the problem separate from the person involved and do not make matters personal.

2. Identify the desired solution or outcome.

3. Schedule a private meeting time with the person involved with the problem.

4. Present the problem as well as detailed examples of the problem. Be specific about events and dates. Include information about how the problem affects the workflow within the office. Ask the other person for input and ideas to help create a solution.

5. Present your own ideas for a solution and then discuss and agree upon a mutual decision to resolve the problem.

are being provoked into a confrontational circumstance, excuse yourself and seek the assistance of your immediate supervisor.

If the problematic situation involves your immediate supervisor, once again try to discuss the matter with him or her in a calm and professional manner. When this is not an option, follow the chain of command within the office. It may be beneficial to request a joint meeting with your supervisor as well as his or her immediate supervisor.

UNPRODUCTIVE COWORKERS **Efficiency** is the heartbeat of a medical office. You may find a fellow coworker slacking on his or her duties and those around left to pick up the pieces. This will cause unwanted stress and pressure for everyone in the office. It is important never to pass judgment on a coworker; oftentimes a change in work behavior is a direct result of a difficult circumstance occurring in the person's personal life.

In most cases it is appropriate to share your concerns with the coworker directly, rather than discussing his or her lack of motivation with other coworkers. It is best to start the conversation in a calm and nonconfrontational manner. You may begin the conversation by saying, "I have some free time, is there anything I can do to help you with your work?" If you know that the coworker is having difficulty organizing tasks, it may be beneficial to begin the conversation by saying, "Please let me know if there is anything that I can do to help you get organized with your work." When situations are beyond your control, once again, it is best to voice your concerns privately with your immediate supervisor.

Above all else, professional medical assistants will not become lax in their duties or mimic the unproductiveness of others.

Sexual Harassment

Sexual harassment is both unwelcome and illegal. Title VII of the Civil Rights Act of 1964 defines *sexual harassment* as follows: "Unwelcome sexual advances, requests for sexual favors, and other verbal or physical conduct of a sexual nature constitutes sexual harassment when submission to or rejection of this conduct explicitly or implicitly affects an individual's employment, unreasonably interferes with an individual's work performance or creates an intimidating, hostile or offensive work environment."[1]

The **U.S. Equal Employment Opportunity Commission** further explains sexual harassment as follows:

- The victim as well as the harasser may be a woman or a man. The victim does not have to be of the opposite sex.
- The harasser can be the victim's supervisor, an agent of the employer, a supervisor in another area, a coworker, or a nonemployee.
- The victim does not have to be the person harassed but could be anyone affected by the offensive conduct.
- Unlawful sexual harassment may occur without economic injury to or discharge of the victim.
- The harasser's conduct must be unwelcome.

---

[1] From http://www.eeoc.gov/types/sexual_harassment.html

Career Tips

Finding useful methods to help with time efficiency is important when working in a busy office. One of the most helpful things for medical assistants to have is a small notepad to carry in their pocket (■ Figure 3-3). This note pad can be used to write down daily task lists, reminders, and helpful hints. At the end of each day, transfer any uncompleted tasks to the top of the next page for the next day. Remember to shred the note paper if it contains any identifying patient information.

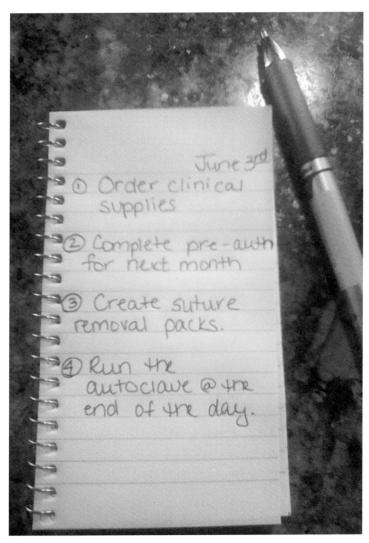

■ FIGURE 3-3

Daily task lists can help the medical assistant with time efficiency.

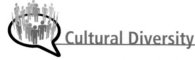

Cultural Diversity

Many European cultures (Italian, French, Spanish, and Greek) much more physically than the American culture. It is not uncommon in these cultures to greet one another with a hug or a kiss on the cheek. While this is acceptable in private encounters, this would not be considered acceptable in public places. In a medical office, the harmless gesture could be misconstrued by some individuals as inappropriate physical contact. The professional medical assistant should always err on the side of caution in regard to physical contact with patients and coworkers.

In addition to obvious unwanted sexual advances, favors, and threats, explicit or inappropriate jokes, emails, pet names, and gestures are also considered forms of sexual harassment. Professional medical assistants should neither participate nor condone this type of behavior. If a person feels he or she is a victim of sexual harassment, he or she must report the offensive behavior to his or her immediate supervisor without haste. Under the law, supervisors have a duty to immediately investigate a claim of sexual harassment. If an investigation results in finding that the accused is guilty of sexual harassment, penalties and punishments are often evoked. Punishments may include suspension or termination from a job. However, in most cases, the employer is held liable for not stopping or preventing the harassment. Therefore, any legal action is generally brought against the employer and not the individual.

Many employers and healthcare organizations are adopting antiharassment policies, which outline the definition and examples of sexual harassment. The state of California was the first state to mandate that supervisors who work for employers with fifty or more employees must attend a two-hour sexual harassment prevention training seminar.

END OF CHAPTER REVIEW

LEARNING OBJECTIVE REVIEW

Complete each learning objective to the best of your ability.

1. Explain the significance of a chain of command within an office environment.

   _____

   _____

   _____

   _____

   _____

2. Describe elements of appropriate workplace conversations.

   _____

   _____

   _____

   _____

   _____

3. Describe how to appropriately address physicians.

   _____

   _____

   _____

   _____

   _____

4. Discuss issues involved with communicating patient information.

   _____

   _____

   _____

   _____

   _____

5. List examples of how to handle various difficult situations in the workplace.

_____

_____

_____

_____

_____

6. Discuss sexual harassment in the workplace.

_____

_____

_____

_____

_____

KEY TERMS

Use each of the following key terms in a sentence that demonstrates your understanding of the word.

1. chain of command:_____

_____

2. compliant:_____

_____

3. confidential:_____

_____

4. efficiency:_____

_____

5. gossip:_____

_____

6. Health Insurance Portability and Accountability Act (HIPAA):_____

_____

7. litigation:_____

_____

8. Office for Civil Rights (OCR):_____

_____

9. practicum:_____

_____

10. sexual harassment:_____

_____

11. supervisor:_____

_____

12. U.S. Department of Health and Human Services:_____

_____

13. U.S. Equal Employment Opportunity Commission_____

_____

CRITICAL THINKING

Reread the workplace scenario at the beginning of the chapter and answer the following questions.

1. According to the information presented in the workplace scenario, would Alicia's conversation with her coworker be considered appropriate?

_____

_____

_____

_____

2. Has anyone in the workplace scenario breached confidential patient information?

_____

_____

_____

_____

3. How do you think Marla would feel after overhearing Alicia's conversation? How should she handle this situation?

_____

_____

_____

_____

DO IT YOURSELF!

Complete the modules below to demonstrate your understanding of the chapter.

Module A

1. Create a chain of command for a medical office with the following employees:
   a. Mary Ann is a clinical medical assistant.
   b. Dr. Jarmaine McWalter owns the medical office.
   c. Ivan works in medical billing and coding.
   d. Sun-Ye is the front desk receptionist.
   e. Jacob is the clinical supervisor.
   f. Jasmine works in the front office doing patient checkout and appointment scheduling.
   g. Avery is the office manager.
   h. Marilyn works as the front office supervisor, overseeing all administrative aspects of the office.
   i. Patrick performs blood draws and administers medications.

Chain of Command

Module B

1. While working as a medical assistant, the physician asks you to make a copy of a patient's medical record. While at the copy machine, a fellow worker is waiting to use the copier. Your coworker begins asking you questions about the patient's file and begins to read the photocopied record. How would you handle this situation?

   _____

   _____

   _____

   _____

   _____

2. You begin to receive sexually explicit emails from a coworker. This coworker has been sending everyone in the office the same emails and thinks that everyone should consider them humorous. What actions would you take in this situation?

   _____

   _____

   _____

   _____

   _____

3. You notice that a coworker removes $10 from the petty cash fund to pay for her lunch that has been delivered from a local deli. She writes "$10 for postage, missing receipt" on the petty cash log. What would you do?

   _____

   _____

   _____

   _____

   _____

4. You work as a clinical medical assistant in a pediatrician's office. Every afternoon, you and a coworker are in charge of working well-baby visits with the physician. This includes providing babies and toddlers with vaccinations and immunizations. This same coworker confides in you that she is addicted to prescription pain medication. She further explains that every day on her afternoon break she will take a combination of Oxycontin and Vicodin "just to make it through the rest of the day." How would you handle this situation?

_____

_____

_____

_____

_____

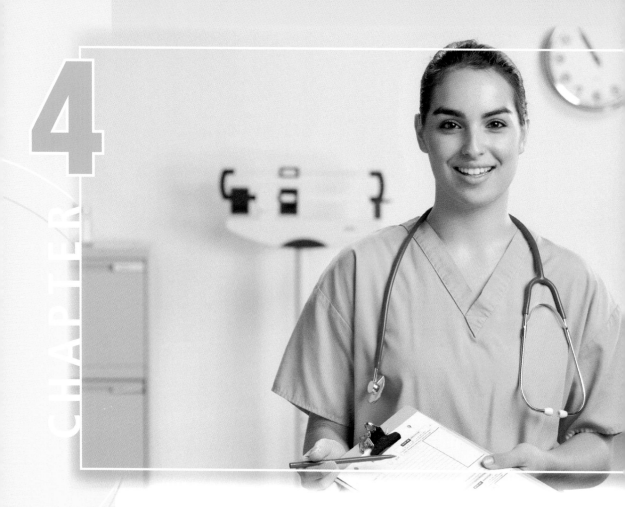

Professionalism with Patients

LEARNING OBJECTIVES

- Explain the importance of customer service within the medical office.
- Identify proper greetings for patients of all ages.
- Describe the pitfalls of using pet names with patients.
- List examples of how professionalism extends into the examination room.
- Identify triggers that could make a patient angry or distraught.
- List the steps in dealing with challenging patients.

Workplace Scenario

Sylvia Gardner is a seventy-two-year-old new patient to Dr. Gosslinger's practice. She has been dropped off for her 9:15 am appointment by a local transportation service for elderly individuals. This same service is scheduled to pick her up from her appointment at 11:15 am. At 10:50 am she is finally taken back to the exam room, and she voices extreme frustration with Marlee, the CMA (AAMA) who is obtaining her vital signs. Sylvia has become so angry that she begins to cry and fears she will miss her transportation service. As Marlee leaves the room, she says to Sylvia, "I'm sorry dear, I am sure the doctor will be right with you."

Introduction

It is possible that the most important concept to understand in regard to professionalism revolves around the area of working with patients. Proper communication, conduct, and respect for patients will form a solid foundation for a professional and mutually beneficial relationship for both the medical assistant and the patient.

Working with Patients

The medical world is in the business of both health services and **customer service**. Excelling at customer service in the medical field involves meeting and exceeding the needs of the patients in the medical office. It involves treating the patient with a level of respect that is not only appreciated but also deserved. The ability to provide quality customer service involves having the quality of being empathetic with patients. **Empathy** simply is the ability to identify and share the feelings of another person. Together, both respect and empathy can create the building blocks for exceptional customer service in the medical field.

Greeting Patients

Medical assistants, more often than not, generally provide the first and lasting impression a patient has of a medical office. This is because the medical assistant is the first medical staff member to spend a significant amount of time with the patient obtaining vital signs and chief complaints. This initial encounter with the patient is exceptionally important as it helps the patient's visit to the office start out on the right foot. A proper greeting can make patients feel valued just as much as an improper greeting can leave them feeling disrespected. One of the most important things to remember when greeting patients is to smile and be sincere. A fake smile or an insincere comment can be taken as sarcastic and rude.

Pet Names

It is never appropriate to use pet names for patients. Some examples of pet names include "honey," "dear," and "hun." Oftentimes, people who use pet names to address others consider them to be terms of endearment. However, such terms can often cause individuals to feel awkward or uncomfortable. Additionally, some cultures may find such terms offensive. This is especially true when "pet" names are addressed to a patient of the opposite sex. It is a good practice to remove these terms from the vocabulary that is used in the medical office. The Career Tips box offers suggestions for appropriate patient greetings based on age and sex.

First Names

Keeping customer service in mind, never address a patient solely by his or her first name. The only exception to this rule is when the medical assistant is calling a patient back into the examination area from the reception area. This helps maintain the patient's privacy among other patients waiting in the reception area. For example, if a medical assistant is ready to bring Mr. Al Jourgensen back to see the doctor, the medical assistant would enter the reception area and say, "Al we are ready for you." When the patient leaves the reception area and is in a private

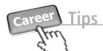

Tips

Proper Greetings

Children

It is appropriate to address patients aged seventeen years or younger by their first name. When a child patient asks you a question, include the child's first name in your response along with a complimentary phrase such as "that is a great question, Sadie."

Adults

When working with adult patients, it is respectful to address them as Mr. or Ms. A. Good tip: when working with female patients, check the demographic sheet of the medical record for marital status (■ Figure 4-1). This will serve as reference regarding which title of courtesy, Miss or Mrs., is appropriate. Addressing elderly patients as Sir or Ma'am demonstrates an often appreciated measure of respect.

■ **FIGURE 4-1**

A medical assistant working with a female patient.

Source: Michal Heron/Pearson Education.

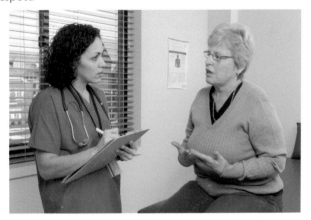

examination room with the medical assistant, the medical assistant should say, "What brings you to the office today, Mr. Jourgensen?" Always addressing a patient on a first name–only basis indicates a certain level of intimacy in a relationship. It is not professional to have that level of intimacy unless specifically directed by the patient. In certain circumstances, patients will prefer to be called by their first name in conversation. When this is the case, make a notation in the patient's chart indicating that the patient prefers to be called by his or her first name. This will serve as a reminder to you and the rest of the staff of the patient's wishes, which ultimately will leave the patient feeling more comfortable and at ease. The Career Tips box offers suggestions for appropriate patient greetings based on age and sex.

In the Examination Room

Professionalism does not stop with a proper greeting and manner of conversation. It extends into the examination room. In the examination room, professionalism is expressed in the form of common **courtesy**. In its simplest form, courtesy is expressing politeness and

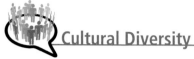

Cultural Diversity

Consider the patient's culture while working in the examination room. Some cultures, particularly Middle Eastern, may require the husband's presence during the examination of his wife. In Asian cultures, many times the female will take on strong nurturing and helping personas. This may translate into a wife wanting to help her husband—for instance, onto an examination table—rather than having the medical assistant be of help. Take verbal and nonverbal cues from patients to identify particular issues of cultural diversity in the examination room.

kindness through attitudes and actions. Often, doctors are running behind, patients are still waiting to be seen half-hour past their appointment time, and minor emergencies are double-booked in an already busy schedule. With all of this going on, medical assistants are under constant pressure to keep up with the fast pace of the office environment. Unfortunately, in such situations the common courtesies of professionalism in the examination room may be missed.

It is in the Details

The patient's main concern when visiting the doctor is to get his or her issues resolved, whether it is monitoring blood pressure or discussing the findings of recent blood tests. Every patient deserves to be treated and cared for as a fellow human being.

■ Table 4-1 provides a list of some often overlooked details. Incorporating these details into the routine within the examination room will not only help patients feel that they are being cared for but also show a level of professionalism through common courtesy.

■ TABLE 4-1 **Important Details to Remember in the Examination Room**

Do	Don't
• Offer a helping hand when the patient steps onto the examination table. This is not only a common courtesy but also a matter of safety.	• Turn your back while the patient attempts to sit on the table.
• Make and maintain eye contact when asking questions regarding chief complaints.	• Keep your eyes glued to the medical chart while asking questions and documenting the responses.
• Offer the patient a magazine or other reading material if the doctor is running behind.	• Tell the patient that the doctor will be right in if he or she is running behind; it is important to be honest.
• Offer a blanket or drape if the patient is in a gown. It may help make the patient feel more comfortable to be covered.	• Assume that the patient is comfortable simply wearing a gown and waiting to be seen.

Handling Uncomfortable Situations

Some patients have anxiety associated with visiting the doctor. Anxieties are heightened when particular procedures must be performed in the office. The procedures that increase anxiety require a certain component of professionalism. They may include the following:

- Physical examinations (particularly for males)
- Gynecological examinations
- Catheterizations
- Sigmoidoscopies
- Breast and testicular examinations
- Hemorrhoidectomies
- Painful procedures such as cryosurgery or ingrown toenail removals

In all cases the most important factors to keep in mind include providing efficient support to the physician and to provide comforting words of support for the patient. Ensure patient privacy by adjusting drapes and lending a helping hand if a positional change is required during the procedure.

Another important factor involved with professionalism is to always be prepared. Preparation applies not only to supplies and equipment used during the procedure but also to the sights, sounds, and smells that happen during the procedure. In the medical office, you must be prepared to see and hear everything. No matter the circumstance, it is important not to make any comments, faces, or gestures that would imply a feeling of shock or disgust. This more advanced concept of professionalism requires practice and skill. Medical assistants must appear both neutral and confidently unconcerned by what is occurring during the medical procedure. The simplest raise of the eyebrows, roll of the eyes, or gasp can make a patient feel embarrassed and uncomfortable. Regardless of the procedure or situation, medical assistants should never pass judgment or belittle the patient but rather should always provide support and advocate on behalf of their patient.

Handling Challenging Patients

While working in the medical field, it is inevitable that at some point you will have to deal with upset, angry, or challenging patients. A wide array of situations or circumstances can cause a patient to become upset. Some common issues that instigate these problems include the following:

- Prolonged wait times
- Medical insurance and billing disputes
- Perceived disrespect toward the patient or a family member
- Emotional or behavioral issues
- News of a grim diagnosis

The ability to handle a difficult patient effectively and to do so with an air of professionalism is an accomplishment that is gained after firsthand experiences. The remainder of this chapter provides some direction for when these circumstances may arise.

■ **FIGURE 4-2**

Medical assistants must remain professional as they attempt to calm angry patients.

Source: Michal Heron/Pearson Education.

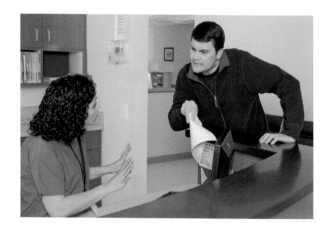

The Angry Patient

As mentioned earlier, a patient can become angry for a variety of reasons. It is important to keep in mind that regardless of the cause of the anger, justified or unjustified, the patient needs to be treated with courtesy. Most medical offices have protocols in place for handling a patient who becomes aggressive. Knowing and understanding the office protocols is a component of professionalism. Should a patient indicate that he or she is going to become verbally or physically abusive, calmly and confidently inform the patient that he or she must leave the medical office at once or the police will be notified. At all costs, attempts should be made to diffuse a situation before it becomes violent. If a patient becomes disorderly, he or she can be a distraction to other patients. In this situation move the disorderly patient to a private room for discussion. Should a patient become **belligerent**—using foul language, being aggressive or violent—it may be necessary to have the patient leave the medical office. Always be cognizant of keeping yourself, other staff members, and other patients safe (■ Figure 4-2).

Consider the following suggestions if you must encounter an angry patient:

- Speak in a calm and even-toned voice. Make gentle eye contact.
- Direct the patient toward a solution regarding his or her problem. Specifically ask, "How may I help resolve this for you?"
- Use reassuring statements that do not assume blame, such as "I understand you are upset. Let's see how we can work this out."
- If necessary, get assistance from an office manager or physician.

It is important to document all encounters with the patient in the medical record. When documenting, provide specific facts regarding the situation and the resolution. Never include personal opinions.

The Emotionally Distraught Patient

Aside from being angry, a patient may become emotionally **distraught**—upset or hysterical—while in the medical office. This often happens when a patient learns the results of medical tests that provide a grim diagnosis. Patients may become upset after any type of loss: death of a loved one, lost job, or recent divorce. Consider the following suggestions when comforting a distraught patient:

- Try to remain composed and express a professional concern. An appropriate response might be "I am so sorry that you are going through this."
- Never tell the patient "I know how you feel." This often will cause the patient to become angry or despondent.
- Offer the patient tissues and a cup of water to help him or her regain composure.
- If resources are available, provide the patient with information regarding support groups.
- Inform the physician of the patient's status before his or her entering the examination room.

It is important to know and understand the medical office protocol for charting such instances. In most cases, some sort of notation will be made in the patient's chart.

END OF CHAPTER REVIEW

LEARNING OBJECTIVE REVIEW

Complete each learning objective to the best of your ability.

1. Explain the importance of customer service within the medical office.

   _____

   _____

   _____

   _____

   _____

2. Identify proper greetings for patients of all ages.

   _____

   _____

   _____

   _____

   _____

3. Describe the pitfalls of using pet names with patients.

   _____

   _____

   _____

   _____

   _____

4. List examples of how professionalism extends into the examination room.

   _____

   _____

   _____

   _____

   _____

5. Identify triggers that could make a patient angry or distraught.

_____

_____

_____

_____

_____

6. List the steps in dealing with challenging patients.

_____

_____

_____

_____

_____

KEY TERMS

Use each of the following key terms in a sentence that demonstrates your understanding of the word.

1. belligerent:_____

_____

2. courtesy:_____

_____

3. customer service:_____

_____

4. distraught:_____

_____

5. empathy:_____

_____

CRITICAL THINKING

Reread the workplace scenario at the beginning of the chapter and answer the following questions.

1. What are some examples of unprofessionalism that are apparent in this scenario?

   _____

   _____

   _____

   _____

2. How should Marlee have handled the issue with Sylvia? Identify some specific action steps that Marlee could have taken.

   _____

   _____

   _____

   _____

3. Explain how the situation with Sylvia becoming angry and upset could have been avoided. What preventative steps should have been taken?

   _____

   _____

   _____

   _____

DO IT YOURSELF!

Complete the modules below to demonstrate your understanding of the chapter.

Module A

Identify a proper greeting for each of the patients listed below.

Patient Information	Proper Greeting
James Hankinson, single male, sixteen years old	
Tanisha Jacobs, married female, twenty-five years old	
Evelyn McCormick, widowed female, sixty-two years old	
Raja Al Adabi, single male, thirty-two years old	
Mario Pecarraro, male, eight years old	
Shirley Johnson, divorced female, thirty-eight years old	
Laurie Branton, single female, nineteen years old	

Module B

With professionalism as the main goal, consider how you would handle the following situations. Explain possible responses and actions.

Scenario 1: Tori Volt, a fifty-one-year-old female patient, has just been diagnosed with malignant melanoma. Her husband is with her in the examination room and he becomes very angry at the diagnosis. He begins to blame her for using tanning beds all these years and for being more concerned about her appearance than her health. The patient is crying.

What would you do?

_____

_____

_____

_____

_____

Scenario 2: Vladimir Golov, a forty-two-year-old male patient, is angry about a bill he has received for $375.00. After some investigation, you find the explanation of benefits from his last visit that shows that he is no longer an active member of the medical insurance plan on file.

What would you do?

_____

_____

_____

_____

_____

Scenario 3: Gemina Rivera, a sixty-four-year-old female patient, has arrived for her 10:30 am appointment. She does not speak English and is scheduled to have an interpreter accompany her to her appointment with the doctor. At 10:55 am the interpreter has not yet arrived for the appointment.

What would you do?

_____

_____

_____

_____

_____

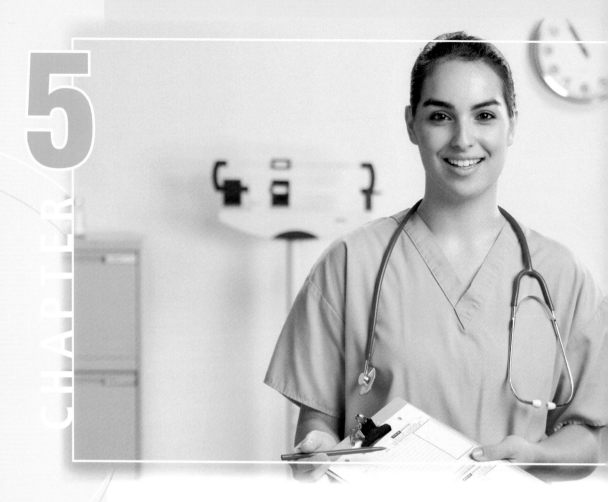

CHAPTER 5

Professionalism and the Medical Record

LEARNING OBJECTIVES

- Explain how professionalism would pertain to medical records.
- List commonalities that pertain to professionalism for both the paper and electronic medical record.
- Describe how charting protocols can relate to professionalism.
- Identify three components of professionalism as it specifically relates to a paper medical record.
- Identify three components of professionalism as it specifically relates to an electronic medical record.

KEY TERMS
conciseness
consistency
defaming
legible
protocol

Workplace Scenario

Santina is a registered medical assistant at a family practice. She is working with Mrs. Lenora Smith, a seventy-eight-year-old patient. There is another patient in the practice, Lenore Smith, who is seventy-six years old. Lenora Smith and Lenore Smith are not relatives. While reviewing Mrs. Lenora Smith's most recent medication list, Santina realizes that the medications listed are not for Lenora Smith as she denies ever using any of the medications listed.

Introduction

Professionalism, as it relates to a medical record, can be a challenging concept to grasp. In most cases, professionalism relates to the manner in which you behave, carry yourself, and interact with others. Therefore, it is difficult to consider how entering information into a record can carry an air of professionalism. Professionalism in maintaining medical records is demonstrated by recognizing and respecting the fact that the medical record is a legal document. Medical assistants will display professionalism by writing thorough and accurate notations with each record.

The Medical Record

Technology is evolving and changing with time; so is the method of maintaining medical records. Today, many medical offices and facilities are doing away with the paper record and converting to electronic medical records. There are models of professionalism that are relevant to both types of records, while other concepts of professionalism are specific to either the paper or the electronic record.

Concepts for Electronic and Paper Medical Records

Medical assisting students are taught the rules and charting methods of medical records throughout their course of study. Because the medical record is considered a legal document, it is important to review the following basic teachings. Having a thorough understanding of documentation guidelines is considered a component of professionalism as it pertains to medical records.

CONSISTENCY AND CONCISENESS The most important rule regarding medical record documentation is the use of **consistency**. *Consistency* refers to a uniform manner in which documentation occurs. The medical office will establish a **protocol** (a manner of performing a procedure) that details charting format, layout, inclusions, and exclusions. The ability to choose proper wording that is well thought and to the point is also an aspect of professionalism. This skill is termed **conciseness**. ■ Figure 5-1 demonstrates the use of concise wording.

Career Tips

Many words or phrases used in medical terminology are abbreviated. However, some medical facilities do not allow the use of all abbreviations. Many medical offices and facilities will have a list of acceptable abbreviations that may be used when charting. It is important, as a part of a professionalism component, to be aware of and use only the medical abbreviations that are allowed by the medical facility where one is employed. Medical offices and facilities, especially accredited institutions, may choose to follow the Official "Do Not Use" List (■ Figure 5-2) that was published by The Joint Commission.

Mary's chief complaint is "I have felt terrible for the past three days." The medical assistant continues to make additional notations in the medical record regarding the patient symptoms. The following exemplifies the difference in concise writing.

Not Concise:

Mary says she has had a fever. She took acetaminophen. She also drank more liquids. After three days her fever was still present.

Concise:

After three days of acetaminophen and increased liquid intake, patient still complains of fever.

■ FIGURE 5-1

An example of how to write a concise chart note.

ITEMS TO AVOID There are certain items that must never be written in the medical record. Just as it is important to know the rules for what must be included in the medical record, it is also necessary to know the items that must always be excluded from the medical record. When charting, it is *never* appropriate to include the following:

- **Defaming** remarks: This includes anything that could be considered insulting or offensive. Example: *Patient appears lazy.*
- Personal opinion: A personal opinion should never be documented. Personal opinions regarding a patient should not be voiced unless they are out of concern for the patient's health. In such an instance, the personal opinion should be voiced in confidence to the patient's physician. Example: *Patient needs to take more showers.*
- Diagnosis: It is outside the medical assistant's scope of practice to diagnose or even to give a hint or a suggestion regarding a possible diagnosis. Such behavior is not only unprofessional but also unethical and illegal. Example: *Patient likely has a urinary tract infection.*

The Paper Medical Record

Many medical offices utilize the paper medical record even though many are transitioning to the electronic medical record. Special considerations must be taken when utilizing paper records.

Writing in the Paper Medical Record

It is important to use clear and **legible** handwriting when writing in the medical record. Legible handwriting refers to that which is neat and easy to read and understand. Unfortunately, the size of lettering is not usually taken into consideration. Handwriting that is too small or

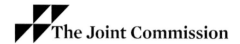

The Joint Commission

Official "Do Not Use" List[1]

Do Not Use	Potential Problem	Use Instead
U (unit)	Mistaken for "0" (zero), the number "4" (four) or "cc"	Write "unit"
IU (International Unit)	Mistaken for IV (intravenous) or the number 10 (ten)	Write "International Unit"
Q.D., QD, q.d., qd (daily)	Mistaken for each other	Write "daily"
Q.O.D., QOD, q.o.d, qod (every other day)	Period after the Q mistaken for "I" and the "O" mistaken for "I"	Write "every other day"
Trailing zero (X.0 mg)* Lack of leading zero (.X mg)	Decimal point is missed	Write X mg Write 0.X mg
MS	Can mean morphine sulfate or magnesium sulfate	Write "morphine sulfate" Write "magnesium sulfate"
MSO$_4$ and MgSO$_4$	Confused for one another	

[1] Applies to all orders and all medication-related documentation that is handwritten (including free-text computer entry) or on pre-printed forms.

*Exception: A "trailing zero" may be used only where required to demonstrate the level of precision of the value being reported, such as for laboratory results, imaging studies that report size of lesions, or catheter/tube sizes. It may not be used in medication orders or other medication-related documentation.

Additional Abbreviations, Acronyms and Symbols
(For <u>possible</u> future inclusion in the Official "Do Not Use" List)

Do Not Use	Potential Problem	Use Instead
> (greater than) < (less than)	Misinterpreted as the number "7" (seven) or the letter "L"	Write "greater than" Write "less than"
	Confused for one another	
Abbreviations for drug names	Misinterpreted due to similar abbreviations for multiple drugs	Write drug names in full
Apothecary units	Unfamiliar to many practitioners	Use metric units
	Confused with metric units	
@	Mistaken for the number "2" (two)	Write "at"
cc	Mistaken for U (units) when poorly written	Write "mL" or "ml" or "milliliters" ("mL" is preferred)
µg	Mistaken for mg (milligrams) resulting in one thousand-fold overdose	Write "mcg" or "micrograms"

Updated 3/5/09

■ FIGURE 5-2

The Official "Do Not Use" List as issued by the Joint Commission. © The Joint Commission, 2012. Reprinted with permission.

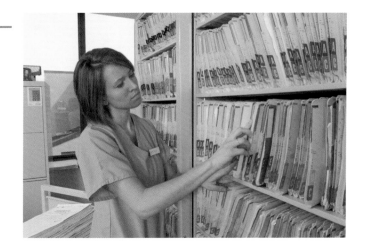

■ FIGURE 5-3

Proper chart filing increases time efficiency in the medical office.

Source: Michal Heron/Pearson Education.

too large may be difficult to read. Also, it may make the entire paper record look inconsistent or even sloppy. Information should be written in the medical record using only black or blue ink; however, many offices use red ink to indicate if a patient has any type of allergies. Follow proper charting guidelines when making a correction in the medical record. Remember, it is never appropriate to scratch out or scribble over an error; rather a simple line drawn through the error with a notation of the correction, date, and initials are adequate for correcting. It is important to note that food and drink should not be present around or near paper medical records. Check the writing surface (table or countertop) for any residue as not to stain the outside of the patient chart. A spill or stain could cause permanent and irrevocable damage to the record.

Locating the Paper Medical Record

A missing or misfiled medical record can be very frustrating and cause delays in treatment and response time. Another component of professionalism, when dealing with paper medical records, is taking the time and consideration to return files to their proper location. Oftentimes, the paper medical record is misplaced due to improper or a complete lack of filing. Taking the extra two or three minutes to correctly file a paper medical record is not only a form of courtesy to others in the medical office who will need to utilize the record at a later point in time, but proper filing is also a way to increase the efficiency of an office by not wasting valuable time searching for a misplaced file (■ Figure 5-3).

OUT GUIDES Some medical offices choose to utilize out guides (■ Figure 5-4) to reduce filing errors. An out guide is placed in the file system when a file is removed to indicate where the file should be returned. Specific notes can be written on the out guide pertaining to who removed the file and the location to where it was moved. Though it takes additional time to place an out

■ FIGURE 5-4

An example of an out guide.

Source: Michal Heron/Pearson Education.

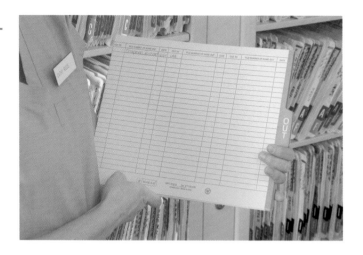

guide in place and make proper notations, proper filing of the medical record could save time in the long run.

PATIENT PRIVACY AND THE PAPER MEDICAL RECORD A key factor of professionalism as it relates to all medical records, paper or electronic, is patient privacy. The Health Insurance Portability and Accountability Act (HIPAA) of 1996 has made patient privacy a legal matter. Medical offices are required to follow the evolving laws that relate to HIPAA and patient privacy. ■ Table 5-1 outlines tips for proper management of patient privacy as it pertains to paper medical records. Understanding and following these tips will help maintain the integrity of patient privacy.

■ TABLE 5-1 **Paper Medical Records: Professionalism through Privacy**

Things to Remember and Check	
• **Is there a signed authorization form?**	• All patients should sign an authorization form indicating those persons authorized to receive information about their health. It is *never* appropriate to assume a family member, spouse, or partner is entitled to this information.
• **Do you have the correct patient chart when filing paperwork and correspondence?**	• Many patients have the same or similar names. When filing information in the paper record, always verify you have the correct patient name. Misfiled patient information is a violation of patient privacy.
• **Did you forget anything on the copy or fax machine?**	• It is easy to forget to remove the original documents from a copy or fax machine. Once the task of copying or faxing has been accomplished, the original documents should be immediately refiled in their proper location.

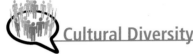

Cultural Diversity

Understanding and respecting diversity among patients must extend to generational diversity. Patients born in earlier generations, such as those born before to the baby boomer generation, may experience hesitation as a medical office becomes more electronically and technologically advanced. Concerns regarding privacy tend to be very real for many of these patients. A medical assistant must be willing to take the time to explain changes and specifically address any patient concerns with patience and care.

The Electronic Medical Record

Technology is always advancing, especially in regard to the medical field. Electronic medical records have become commonplace in hospitals and large medical facilities. Individual medical practices, especially those associated with hospitals and larger medical facilities, are now implementing electronic medical records (■ Figure 5-5) to replace the paper medical record. As more and more offices convert to electronic medical records, various aspects of professionalism regarding the electronic medical record will need to be taken into consideration.

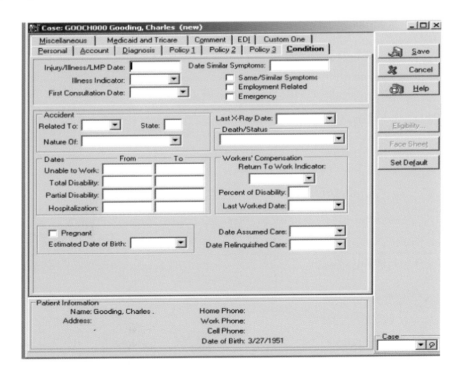

■ FIGURE 5-5

The electronic medical record allows for time-efficient data entry. Reprinted with permission from Medicomp.

User Knowledge

Medical offices and facilities that utilize electronic medical records will recognize and admit to a learning curve associated with the conversion of the paper medical record to the electronic medical record. Companies that have developed various electronic medical record software systems often conduct both in-office and out-of-office training sessions. Each member of the medical office team is responsible for learning, understanding, and implementing the software system. Attending seminars, taking detailed notes, knowing the vendor representative for the medical office, understanding how to contact technical support, and proper maintenance of electronic medical record systems are components of professionalism as it relates to electronic medical records.

PATIENT PRIVACY AND THE ELECTRONIC MEDICAL RECORD The considerations of privacy, as it relates to patient information, are taken to a higher level when the electronic medical record is used. Many software systems implement automatic safety protocols to help protect the privacy and integrity of the electronic medical record. Some of these protocols include the following:

- Individual user names and passwords: Each person in the office is provided a unique user name and password. Often, the user's password is required to be changed on a regular basis to maintain security.
- Restricted access: Certain components of the medical record will be restricted to only those who are authorized or have clearance to view it.
- Automatic logoff: If a user has logged into a medical record but the record has remained stagnant for a predetermined amount of time, the software system will automatically log out the user and enter into a secure mode.

■ Table 5-2 outlines tips for proper management of patient privacy as it pertains to electronic medical records. New laws regarding HIPAA compliance as it relates to electronic data are also included in the table.

■ TABLE 5-2 **Electronic Medical Records: Professionalism through Privacy**

Things to Remember and Check	
• **Keep your login ID and password protected.**	• Do not keep your login ID and password information where it can be easily accessed.
• **Make sure you have the correct medical record.**	• Triple-check that you are entering information into the correct patient medical record. Entering information into the wrong record is a privacy issue.
• **Stay abreast of current privacy legislation as it relates to the electronic exchange of patient information.**	• Legislations such as the The Health Information Technology for Economic and Clinical Health (HITECH) Act and HIPAA 5010 have initiated changes in the way electronic medical records are implemented as well as how electronic patient data is exchanged.

END OF CHAPTER REVIEW

LEARNING OBJECTIVE REVIEW

Complete each learning objective to the best of your ability.

1. Explain how professionalism would pertain to medical records.

   _____

   _____

   _____

   _____

   _____

2. List commonalities that pertain to professionalism for both the paper and electronic medical record.

   _____

   _____

   _____

   _____

   _____

3. Describe how charting protocols can relate to professionalism.

   _____

   _____

   _____

   _____

   _____

4. Identify three components of professionalism as it specifically relates to a paper medical record.

   _____

   _____

   _____

   _____

5. Identify three components of professionalism as it specifically relates to an electronic medical record.

_____

_____

_____

_____

_____

KEY TERMS

Use each of the following key terms in a sentence that demonstrates your understanding of the word.

1. conciseness:_____

_____

2. consistency:_____

_____

3. defaming:_____

_____

4. legible:_____

_____

5. protocol:_____

_____

CRITICAL THINKING

Reread the workplace scenario at the beginning of the chapter and answer the following questions.

1. According to the information presented in the workplace scenario, what likely happened to the medication list? How could professionalism have played a role to prevent this error?

_____

_____

_____

_____

2. Santina notices a strong odor coming from Mrs. Lenora Smith. Based on her appearance, it would seem as if she is not bathing on a regular basis. How should Santina address this issue; what would she write in the medical record?

_____

_____

_____

_____

3. A week after Mrs. Lenora Smith's appointment, she requests to have a prescription for a shower chair faxed to a local durable medical equipment company. The doctor okays the request. What are some precautions, as they relate to patient privacy, Santina should take to accomplish this task?

_____

_____

_____

_____

DO IT YOURSELF!

Complete the modules below to demonstrate your understanding of the chapter.

Module A

Below are some statements that must be rewritten to be more concise. Considering professionalism, rewrite the statements as if you would be entering them in a paper medical record. Use medical abbreviations, when possible. There are no exclusions regarding abbreviations.

1. Patient complains of upset stomach. Patient complains of vomiting. Patient complains of a fever over 101.00, constantly over the past three days.

_____

_____

_____

_____

2. While walking her dog in Central Park, Meghan (the patient) tripped over a piece of broken concrete that had fallen from an overhead bridge. She has had ankle pain for the past five days. Went to the emergency room two days ago and an X-ray showed no fracture. The medication prescribed in the emergency room has not been very helpful.

_____

_____

_____

_____

3. Patient contracted chlamydia from previous girlfriend. Patient's parents are unaware that he is sexually active. Patient is nineteen years old and would like to ensure that his health information is going to be kept private from his parents. He would like to be treated for the sexually transmitted disease and pay for the treatment out of this own pocket, rather than have it submitted to medical insurance.

_____

_____

_____

_____

4. A seven-year-old female patient presents to the office with a possible case of head lice. The mother is concerned because there was a lice outbreak at her child's day care. The daughter does not seem to be itching all that much, but the mother insists that she saw "eggs" in her daughter's hair. The mother described the eggs as "little tiny white seeds that wouldn't come off." The daughter is worried that her friends at school are going to make fun of her if she does have lice.

_____

_____

_____

_____

5. A forty-five-year-old male is complaining about problems with sleep. He states he is "hav-ing headaches every morning when he wakes up." He also includes, "I drive my wife crazy with my snoring; in fact, she won't even sleep in the same room as me. It is just terrible because I can't sleep, I am always tired, and then I wake up with a headache. Something has to change."

_____

_____

_____

_____

Module B

Staying aware of current legislations and issues pertaining to patient privacy is a component of pro-fessionalism. Utilize an Internet search engine to find the answers to the following questions:

1. What is the HITECH Act? Summarize your findings.

_____

_____

_____

_____

_____

_____

_____

_____

2. What is HIPAA 5010? What are the phases of implementation?

_____

_____

_____

_____

_____

_____

_____

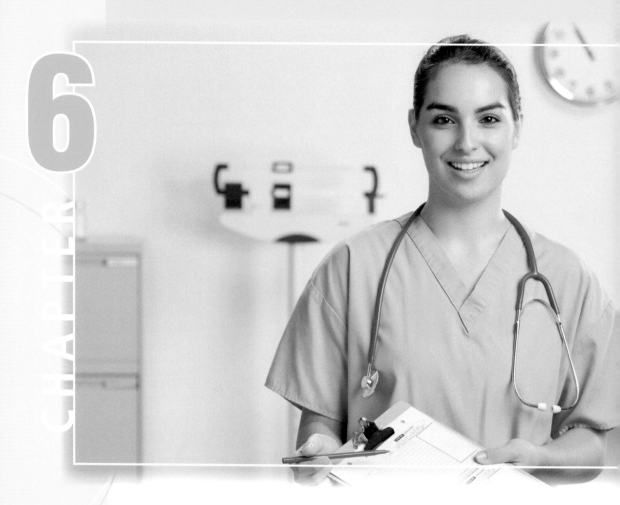

CHAPTER

Professionalism for Administrative Medical Assisting

LEARNING OBJECTIVES

- Identify and explain two of the eight traits of proper telephone etiquette.

- List qualities that would be required to maintain a professional image and create a positive first impression.

- Explain how professionalism may be attributed to billing procedures.

- Name two ways patient information can be guarded when gathering patient information from a new or existing patient.

- Explain the roles of maintaining confidentiality and time efficiency as components of professionalism when coordinating the release of medical information.

KEY TERMS
efficacy
personal impression

Workplace Scenario

Meredith has recently changed positions with Pearson Physicians Group. Instead of working as a clinical administrative assistant, she is now working in the front office as an administrative medical assistant. She is hoping to broaden her skill set and refine skills she has not used since her days of externship. During her training in the front office, she will be working with Jenny. Jenny, a registered medical assistant, has worked in the front office for over five years and is known to be highly knowledgeable in her job.

Introduction

Professionalism is of the utmost importance when working within the realms of administrative medical assisting. Oftentimes, it is an administrative medical assistant who has the opportunity to provide a patient with his or her first impression of a medical office. This occurs when the administrative medical assistant is greeting a first-time patient at the front desk or answering the telephone when a new patient calls the office. The conduct and professionalism of the staff members in a medical office provide not only a first impression but also a lasting impression. It is essential, through proper professionalism, that patients hold the medical office in high esteem from their very first encounter.

Professionalism in the Tasks of the Administrative Medical Assistant

Administrative medical assistants often have the most interaction with patients. Consider the following list of tasks often performed by an administrative medical assistant:

- Telephone interactions including scheduling and taking messages for the physician
- Greeting and registering of new and existing patients at the front desk
- Execution of billing procedures by collecting and posting payments

All of these tasks require excellent communication skills and an understanding of the importance that professionalism plays when interacting with patients. Proficient professionalism not only benefits the patient but also contributes to the well-being of the medical office.

Telephone Interactions

Whether it is scheduling an appointment, taking a message, or providing assistance, the telephone will play a commanding role in the interactions between the patient and a medical office (■ Figure 6-1). Many traits of proper telephone etiquette have been taught in textbooks; however,

■ FIGURE 6-1

Medical assistants practicing proper telephone etiquette will make the patient feel at ease. *Source:* Michal Heron/Pearson Education.

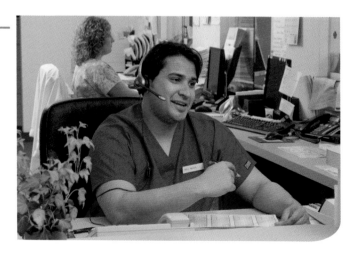

■ TABLE 6-1 **Telephone Etiquette Skills**

Etiquette Skill

- Answer the telephone by the third ring.
- Never allow a caller to wait on hold longer than thirty seconds without returning to the call.
- Smile when you speak; it helps portray a positive attitude.
- Be sincere; a caller can sense insincerity.
- Always state your name to the caller.
- If applicable, provide an estimated time frame for a return call.
- Never interrupt someone while he or she is speaking; always allow the person to finish his or her sentence or thought.
- End a telephone call with a polite and courteous closing such as "Thank you for calling" or "Have a nice day."

the importance of the matter justifies repeating. ■ Table 6-1 reinforces the skills of proper telephone etiquette. These skills should be demonstrated with every telephone interaction.

Give thought to words that are spoken and remain sincere. Consider the difference in the following greetings:

- "Pearson Physicians Group, this is Suzy. Can I help you?"
- "Thank you for calling Pearson Physicians Group, this is Suzy. How may I help you?"

The second greeting sounds more warm and welcoming to the caller. When a caller feels welcomed and well taken care of, he or she tends to be more cooperative and polite.

Additionally, in some instances it is very important to use caution when speaking with patients over the phone. ■ Table 6-2 provides specific circumstances where caution should be used as well as appropriate responses. A general rule to follow is never make promises or ensure outcomes that are out of your control.

■ TABLE 6-2 **Speaking with Caution**

Scenario	Do Not Say	Instead, Say
A patient is calling about wanting to change her blood pressure medication.	"The doctor will call you back about this matter."	"Someone from the office will be returning your call after the doctor has reviewed your request."
A patient is calling about the results of her blood work.	"I am sure the results were fine if you haven't heard anything yet."	"We will call you with your results after the doctor has had a chance to review them."
A patient is calling and is angry about an insurance error.	"I am sure we can get that fixed."	"I understand your frustration. Let me look into this and see if there is a solution."
A patient is calling to find out if his insurance company provided authorization for a procedure.	"I am not sure; I will call you back later."	"I will need to look into this. I will call you back by the end of the working day and let you know what I find out."

Career Tips

Rarely is importance placed on the interaction between medical offices and fellow peers. When speaking with staff members at another medical office or medical facility, the same amount of professionalism and courtesy should be bestowed as if one were speaking with a patient. Opinions regarding the professionalism of other medical offices are quickly established during phone calls regarding mutual patients.

Personal Impressions

A front-desk medical assistant plays a vital role in the patient's perception of a medical office as it is this individual who will provide the initial, **personal impression** of the facility. A personal impression is a lasting mental image that reflects a person's interactions, encounters, and overall view of an event. Medical office managers often choose the person responsible for registration and greeting very carefully. *Sincere, cheerful, helpful, patient,* and *organized* are all adjectives that should describe the person chosen for this very important position within the office. Patients will view an administrative medical assistant who has a polished sense of professionalism as approachable and willing to help.

Some may view the tasks of greeting and registering patients as mundane; however, these duties will often dictate not only the patient's perception of the office but also the **efficacy**, or the efficiency and effectiveness, of billing and payments for services. The front-desk administrative medical assistant will verify the patient's address, birth date, and medical insurance provider on file with the medical office. Failure to update this important information can result in unnecessary payment delays.

KEEPING UP APPEARANCES The medical office should always remain neat and orderly, particularly in areas where patients will be spending a lot of time, for instance the reception area or examination room. While a patient is waiting in the reception area or to see the doctor, he or she often has little else to do other than look around. The condition and appearance of these areas help patients form opinions about the office. Areas that are dirty or cluttered will cause patients to think that the office is not properly cleaned or being cared for. This can then translate to an overall opinion that the practice and those who work there are not professional.

The reception area should appear bright and clean. Clutter and garbage should be cleaned up throughout the day. Desks should remain tidy and organized, not overcrowded with pictures, personal items, or knickknacks. Office decorations, of any sort, should remain tasteful and understated. Examination rooms should be cleaned after every patient, including wiping or disinfecting the examination table, changing paper, and making sure any garbage is placed in the trash receptacle.

Billing Procedures

Administrative medical assistants are also given the responsibility of performing billing and collection procedures. In such cases, the role of professionalism is often understated and overlooked. Professionalism for billing and collections is demonstrated in the following traits:

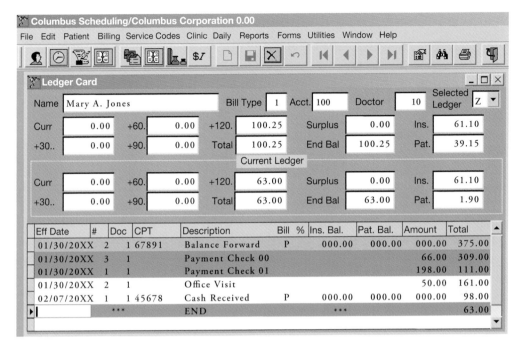

FIGURE 6-2

Administrative medical assistants utilize billing software to keep patient accounts up-to-date.

- Organization: When submitting claims and posting payments, it is essential to keep important information including the medical chart, explanation of benefits, and payment receipts in a neat and organized fashion. This will help if a question regarding a billing procedure should ever arise. Additionally, clearly written and concise notes pertaining to specific patient situations should be included within the organized paperwork.
- Punctuality: Claims should be filed as soon as possible following the date of service. Likewise, posting payments should be done immediately on receipt. This ensures that patient accounts are kept up-to-date (■ Figure 6-2).
- Politeness: It is inevitable that a medical assistant will need to discuss benefits and coverage-related issues with customer or provider service departments of medical insurance companies. While it is important to state the issue at hand in a clear and concise manner, remaining polite while conveying any concerns will result in a more positive and beneficial outcome. It is a serious misconception that excessive firmness or a harsh tone is necessary when trying to achieve a desired result. On the contrary, politeness and kindness have proved to be more effective tools for patient advocacy regarding medical insurance issues.

Professionalism through Patient Confidentiality

Patient confidentiality is a matter that must be adhered to by all members of a medical team. As discussed earlier in this chapter, the administrative medical assistant will interact most frequently with patients and therefore must be acutely aware of adhering to the utmost degree of professionalism when dealing with patient confidentiality.

Gathering Patient Information

Scheduling a patient appointment and greeting patients in the medical office will require an exchange of personal and confidential patient information. When speaking on the phone with a patient, it is important to repeat specific information back to the patient to verify accuracy. When doing so, the administrative medical assistant should speak in a quiet or hushed voice in order to prevent others around him or her from overhearing. If applicable, it is ideal for this information to be obtained in a separate location away from the general office. Some offices provide a sliding glass window that separates the front office from the reception area. In these cases, the window should always remain closed except when interacting with individual patients in the reception area.

The same is true when a patient is providing information upon arriving for his or her appointment. Any exchange of personal and private information should be done in an area out of earshot of other people in the office. The best practice is to have the patient enter a separate and private area for registration. Unfortunately, not all offices have the space for a separate registration area. Again, in such instances, it is important to speak in a quiet tone ensuring that others cannot hear the exchange of information. Although it may seem redundant to discuss these matters and how they should be handled, remember that patient confidentiality is a matter of not only professionalism but also the law, according to HIPAA (Health Insurance Portability and Accountability Act).

Requests for Health Information

Most medical offices strictly adhere to their HIPAA confidentiality policies regarding the request of patient health information. The request for a patient's health information is very common in the medical office and the purposes for the requests vary greatly. Regardless of the

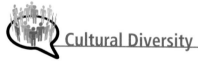

Cultural Diversity

The United States and many Western cultures place a large emphasis on eye contact. It may be considered rude or a sign of insecurity when someone does not look at a person directly in the eye while speaking. Eastern countries, such as Japan, have a different perception of eye contact. In many eastern Asian cultures, maintaining direct eye contact is a sign of disrespect. This must be considered when communicating with patients from other cultures. Taking note of both verbal and nonverbal cues, along with valuing cultural differences, will help medical assistants understand patients and their communication styles.

reason, the medical assistant's role regarding professionalism in the release of health information is to maintain patient confidentiality, process requests in a timely manner, and adhere to all office policies.

MAINTAINING CONFIDENTIALITY When performing the task of releasing health information, it is necessary to ensure that proper steps are being taken to protect the patient's privacy. First, it is necessary to double-check that you are releasing information for the correct patient. The typical release of information form (see ■ Figure 6-3 for an example) will include the patient's name and date of birth. Match this against the medical chart that has been pulled to fulfill the request. Second, it is important to release *only that* medical information that falls within the specified date range indicated on release form. Finally, make sure that the patient has signed the release form and that it has been witnessed. This release form will become a part of the patient's permanent medical record and must be treated as a legal document.

TIME MATTERS All release of information requests should be processed as soon as possible. Again, maintaining efficiency in this regard reflects on one's professionalism. Many requests will be required for a consultation appointment with a specialist; therefore, punctual processing will ensure that the patient's information will be received by the specialist's office before to the patient's appointment.

Many offices will utilize fax machines to ensure that information reaches the intended individual or office quickly. Although this is a great instrument for time efficiency, it is important that the information transmitted via fax is received by the correct individual. All faxes should include a HIPAA-compliant fax cover sheet. A compliant fax cover sheet will include a disclaimer indicating that information should be destroyed if it is not received by the intended recipient. The following exemplifies the wording of a disclaimer statement:

> *Confidentiality Notice: This fax is intended only for use by the addressee(s) named herein and may contain legally privileged and/or confidential information. If you are not the intended recipient of this fax (or the person responsible for delivering this document to the intended recipient), you are hereby notified that any dissemination, distribution, printing, or copying of this email, and any attachment thereto, is strictly prohibited. If you have received this fax in error, please respond to the individual sending the fax, and permanently delete all printed information.*

ADHERING TO OFFICE POLICIES AND PROCEDURES Office policies and procedures will vary by office. However, it is essential that the policies and procedures involved are followed closely by all staff members responsible for releasing a patient's health information. Unfortunately, bad habits can be formed by using shortcuts in office protocol. Again, it cannot be overemphasized that adhering to all safeguards relating to a patient's privacy regarding health information is a matter of not only professionalism but also legality.

PEARSON PHYSICIANS GROUP

Shaina McWalter, D.O.
123 Michigan Avenue
Parker Heights, IL 60610
(312) 123-1234

RELEASE OF MEDICAL RECORDS

TODAY'S DATE:_____

PATIENT NAME: _____

PATIENT DATE OF BIRTH: _____/_____/_____

I hereby authorize and request that you release to

_____
(Doctor Name)

_____
(Address, City, State, ZIP)

All medical records in your possession concerning any examination, diagnosis, and/or treatment rendered to me during the period from
_____ to _____.

_____
Signature of Patient, Legal Guardian, or Power of Attorney

_____
(Relationship)

_____
Witness Signature

■ FIGURE 6-3

An example of a medical release of information.

Succeeding as an Administrative Medical Assistant

Administrative medical assistants who demonstrate exemplary professionalism skills will more likely be promoted to positions with greater responsibility over others who lack professionalism. Administrative medical assistants may be promoted to an area supervisor, an office or practice manager, or even positions within recruiting and human resources. Although some of these positions may require that the medical assistant obtain additional training or schooling, there are opportunities everywhere for bright and engaging employees.

Employees are often judged on how they perform their job. One of the least professional employees could say, "That is not in my job description, so I am not going to do it." This point of view will ensure that the employee will not move up the career ladder as it practically shows unprofessionalism. They will be viewed as lacking teamwork, unmotivated, and possibly lazy. A professional would view an additional task as a challenge to be met, striving to find a solution, and a possible opportunity to engage in teamwork to accomplish a task. These are personal qualities that are highly sought after and with practice, attainable by many people.

END OF CHAPTER REVIEW

LEARNING OBJECTIVE REVIEW

Complete each learning objective to the best of your ability.

1. Identify and explain two of the eight traits of proper telephone etiquette.

    _____

    _____

    _____

    _____

    _____

2. List qualities that would be required to maintain a professional image and create a positive first impression.

    _____

    _____

    _____

    _____

    _____

3. Explain how professionalism may be attributed to billing procedures.

    _____

    _____

    _____

    _____

    _____

4. Name two ways patient information can be guarded when gathering patient information from a new or existing patient.

    _____

    _____

    _____

    _____

    _____

5. Explain the roles of maintaining confidentiality and time efficiency as components of professionalism when coordinating the release of medical information.

_____

_____

_____

_____

_____

KEY TERMS

Use each of the following key terms in a sentence that demonstrates your understanding of the word.

1. efficacy:_____

_____

2. personal impression:_____

_____

CRITICAL THINKING

Reread the workplace scenario at the beginning of the chapter and answer the following questions.

1. Meredith has received a call from Dr. Watson's office. Joy, the medical assistant calling from Dr. Watson's office, is requesting copies of recent lab results regarding a mutual patient. Meredith explains to Joy that the patient must sign a release of information prior to her sending the lab work. Joy, rather curtly, informs Meredith that because of the close relationship between Dr. Watson and Pearson Physicians Group, many times the necessity for the release of information has been overridden. Joy adds that the patient has an appointment at their office in two hours and they need the lab results before the appointment. How should Meredith handle this situation?

_____

_____

_____

_____

2. Meredith receives a call from Mrs. Erin Angelotti. Mrs. Angelotti is wondering if her health insurance company has provided preauthorization for an overnight sleep study that is scheduled for tomorrow night at Memorial Hospital. Upon investigating the matter, Meredith learns that the insurance company was never contacted regarding this issue. What would be the most professional way to handle this circumstance?

_____

_____

_____

_____

3. While working in the front office, Meredith observes Jenny open the reception window and say to the patient sitting across the room, "Mr. Jeffrey, did your insurance change when you lost your job?" Meredith is shocked by what happened. What should Jenny have done differently? Does Meredith have any grounds for approaching Jenny about the incident?

_____

_____

_____

_____

DO IT YOURSELF!

Complete the modules below to demonstrate your understanding of the chapter.

Module A

Indicate a proper and professional response to the following comments:

Patient Comment	Your Action/Response
"Dr. McWalter promised me free samples of my medication." • The patient has just called you on the phone.	
"Your office told me this procedure would be covered by my insurance. If you think I am paying this bill, you are crazy." • The patient has approached the front desk and is speaking in a loud tone.	
"I want my medical record now, so that I do not ever have to come back to this office." • The office policy is that any copies of a patient's medical record require forty-eight-hours' notice.	

Module B

Indicate, by placing items in numerical order, which tasks of the administrative medical assistant should be completed first. Give a brief explanation regarding your answers. Keep in mind that time management is a key component of professionalism.

_____ Follow up with a telephone message from a prospective new patient regarding medical insurance coverage.

Explanation: _____

_____

_____ Complete a request for the release of medical information for a patient who is moving next month to a different state.

Explanation: _____

_____

_____ Deal with an upset patient in the waiting room.

Explanation: _____

_____

_____ Complete a request for the release of medical information for a five-year-old patient who is starting kindergarten in two days and requires immunization records for admittance into school.

Explanation: _____

_____

_____ Make copies of new patient welcome packets to replenish the stock on hand.

Explanation: _____

_____

_____ Post billing and insurance payments that were received in the mail today.

Explanation: _____

_____

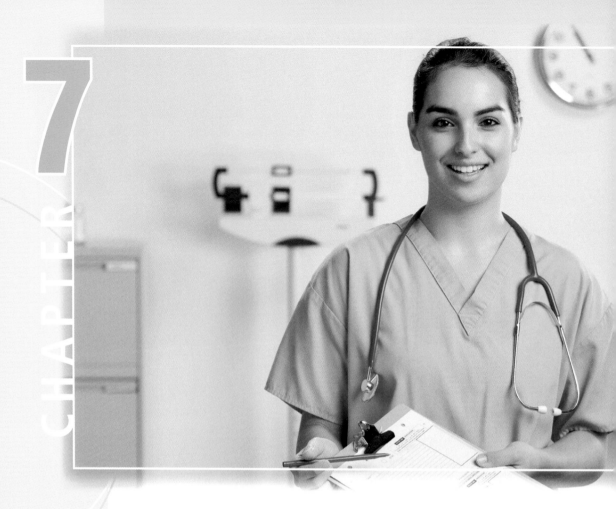

CHAPTER 7

Professionalism in Communication

LEARNING OBJECTIVES

- Explain how communication barriers can affect the role of professionalism in the medical office.

- Describe tools that are available to assist with patients who have a language barrier.

- List particular considerations that should be taken into account when communicating with visually and hearing-impaired patients.

- Identify at least three top priorities when handling an emotional patient, and why they are important.

- Name two roles professionalism plays when dealing with written correspondence.

- Summarize rules for email usage in the medical office.

KEY TERMS
active descriptions
barrier
bilingual
correspondence
decorum
intricacies
refugee
transcribe

Workplace Scenario

Sylvia Oktenburg has arrived for her scheduled appointment with Dr. McWalters. The appointment schedule indicates that she was scheduled to see Dr. McWalters for extreme pain in her lower left quadrant. Mrs. Oktenburg has complete hearing loss in both of her ears. Her translator is now ten minutes late for the appointment and Mrs. Oktenburg is becoming visibly upset. Talisha, Dr. McWalters's medical assistant, is beginning to panic because Dr. McWalters is already running late on her schedule.

Introduction

The backbone of professionalism, as it relates to every component of the medical office, is communication. Earlier chapters have touched on the importance of various forms of communication including greeting new patients, speaking on the telephone, and making notations in the medical record. This chapter takes a more in-depth look at the importance of communication and the manner in which one should communicate with various patient groups and other medical professionals.

The Role of Communication

Communication has vastly changed over the years. As technology constantly develops and evolves, new forms of communication will integrate into everyone's daily lives. This will infiltrate into the medical arena as new forms of communication between patients and other medical professionals become available. However, still, there are core concepts of communication as it relates to professionalism that will never change regardless of the advancements in technology. Some of these concepts include maintaining a positive image, being courteous, and respecting the patient.

Communication Barriers

A **barrier** is simply an obstacle that must be overcome. It is necessary to emphasize that a barrier is not social stigma, or a problem that must be fixed. Communication barriers are unavoidable in the medical arena. The professional medical assistant will recognize a communication barrier and formulate a plan to communicate effectively in spite of the barrier. Realizing the correct plan of communication may take some time and will often result after trial and error, strategic planning, and group effort.

Examples of common communication barriers often found in the medical office include the following:

- Language barrier: Patients who do not speak English as their primary language
- Special needs barrier: Patients who have visual, hearing, or learning impairments
- Emotional barrier: Patients who are saddened, anxious, or ill-tempered

Each of these examples will be discussed in rest of the chapter.

Professionalism in Multicultural Communication

The United States of America has a very high number of immigrants from a vast number of countries throughout the world. It is because of this that the United States has been termed the *melting pot*. Although the United States is one nation, it is comprised of individuals from different countries, customs, and religions.

Medical assistants work with a variety of patients from a multitude of cultures and personal beliefs. Professionally speaking, it is important to understand the major dynamics of cultures, specifically in regard to personal interaction and communication. It is impossible, however,

■ TABLE 7-1 **Tips for Cross-Cultural Communication**

Tip	Take Note
Speak slowly	If English is not the patient's primary language, slow your speech. Speak slower than normal, but in a respectable and intelligible voice.
Ask individual questions	Take time with communication. Rather than asking a patient "What medications are you taking; do you need any refills?" Ask each question individually, allowing the patient to respond appropriately and making the patient not feel rushed.
Write down information	Important information, including instructions or directions, should be clearly written. If handwriting is illegible, type the directions or instructions using word-processing software.
Reaffirm information	After a patient has shared information, summarize and repeat the information back to the patient. This will ensure that everything has been understood correctly.
Avoid slang terms	Avoid misunderstandings by deleting slang terms from your vocabulary. Slang terms can cause confusion even to a person who speaks English as his or her second language fluently. For instance, rather than saying "What's up?" say "How are you doing?"
Cut out the humor	Many cultures take business and healthcare very seriously. It is often a sign of disrespect to make jokes about important matters.
Maintain propriety	When there is doubt or lack of experience with a patient from a particular cultural sect, err on the side of caution. Always choose taking a conservative approach to communication.

to learn and understand the **intricacies**, or details, of every culture that is represented in the United States. When working in an office with a high number of cross-cultural patients, it is a good rule to learn the beliefs and customs of the culture of people with whom you will have the most interaction. ■ Table 7-1 includes generalities that should be taken into consideration when dealing with a cross-cultural population. These tips can be applied when working with any person whose culture or language is different from yours.

Dealing with Language Barriers

It is very likely that the medical assistant will encounter a patient who does not speak or understand English. Many of these patients will bring family members or professional interpreters along with them to every appointment. In such cases it is important to make a notation in

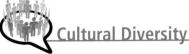

Cultural Diversity

Religion plays different roles in terms of cultural diversity. A person's religious views may shape his or her approach to medicine, treatment, and even choosing a provider. It is not appropriate to ever broaden or generalize a patient based upon your presumption of his or her religious views. Every patient should be valued and cared for regardless of religion or creed. In turn, it is not acceptable to share or discuss your own personal religious beliefs with patients as this can often make them feel uncomfortable. The medical office must be viewed as an establishment of tolerance and acceptance.

the patient's chart indicating that the patient is non-English speaking. Also, make note of the name and phone number of the patient's family member or translator who will accompany the patient to his or her appointments.

Spanish is the second most spoken language in the United States. There is a high demand for medical assistants who are **bilingual**, those who fluently speak more than one language, in English and Spanish. Medical assistants who are not bilingual and live in an area with a high Spanish-speaking population should learn key Spanish phrases. Additionally, it is helpful to have a Spanish-English dictionary or electronic translator. Free translation services are also available on the Internet, for example, www.freetranslation.com, www.translate.google.com, and www.wordlingo.com.

Understanding how to help a patient, quick problem solving, and knowing how to utilize community resources is another aspect of professionalism through multicultural communication. Information regarding agencies that could provide assistance, including emergency translation services, should be readily available. Some of these agencies may include social service agencies, the Office for Civil Rights, and private **refugee**, or immigrant, foundations.

Professionalism and the Special Needs Patient

Patients with special needs may require additional variations or forms of communication. It is essential to remember to treat patients with special needs with the same respect and **decorum**, dignity, and politeness as you would treat any other patient. The professional medical assistant should treat special needs patients in the same manner as other patients, while at the same time recognizing the various aspects that are needed to modify or improve communication with special needs patients.

Communicating with the Visually Impaired

Verbal communication is especially important when working with the visually impaired patient. The professional medical assistant will always, first, ask the patient how he or she can be of assistance. It is never appropriate to assume the form or degree of assistance a special needs patient will require. Many visually impaired patients appreciate **active descriptions** and explanations. Active descriptions will be used to explain the patient's surrounding as well as detail procedures that are being performed. Box 7-1 includes examples of active descriptions.

Visually impaired patients might often be assisted by a service animal. Service animals have been specially trained to help patients with disabilities, including the visually impaired, to help guide and protect them. Service animals are to be viewed as working animals and not pets. Therefore, it is not appropriate to pet or playfully interact with service animals.

Additionally, assistive mechanisms including white canes can help in aiding those with visual impairments. White canes are long, slender, and handheld that extend in front of the visually impaired individual. The individual will use the cane in a *tapping* motion, often from side to side. When a patient has become situated in an examination room, ask the patient if he or she would like to hold onto the cane during the examination or if he or she would like it to be placed someplace specifically.

BOX 7-1 Active Descriptions for Visually Impaired Patients

Situation	An active description for the situation
• Escorting a patient to an examination room	"Mr. Jefferson, we will be heading down this narrow hall to the examination room that is about seven feet ahead of us on the right-hand side."
• Obtaining a blood pressure reading	"Mr. Jefferson, I am going to take your blood pressure now. I am going to place the cuff on your arm above your elbow. Now, I will begin to inflate the cuff. It will feel tight for a few moments and then it will begin to deflate."
• Assisting the patient onto an examination table	"Mr. Jefferson, now that Dr. McWalters is in the examination room, I would like to have you sit on the exam table. How can I best assist you? Would you like to hold onto my arm for guidance?"

Communicating with the Hearing-Impaired Patient

Communication with hearing-impaired patients is often viewed as more challenging. The reason for this, however, is due to the lack of information and understanding on behalf of those attempting to communicate with the hearing impaired. A medical assistant with a professional disposition will understand that communicating with the hearing impaired simply requires more time, planning, and patience.

Most hearing-impaired patients utilize American Sign Language to communicate. American Sign Language utilizes the hands and arms to create gestures and movements to communicate during conversation. It would be appropriate for any medical office to have on hand a copy of the American Sign Language alphabet and numbers. This will enable the medical professionals to communicate with the hearing-impaired patients, even through signing the individual letters of ■ Figure 7-1 illustrates the American Sign Language alphabet.

Consider the following tips when communicating with the hearing-impaired patient:

- **Always speak directly to the patient:** Oftentimes, patients will bring interpreters along with them to medical appointments and examinations. The interpreter may be a professional or a family member who is trained in the use of sign language. When speaking with the patient, always direct conversation to the patient and not the interpreter. To do otherwise is a sign of disrespect and lack of knowledge.
- **Do not shout:** Many times shouting or speaking excessively loud will not enable the patient to hear any clearer: and it can cause the patient to shut down emotionally or become embarrassed.

SIGN LANGUAGE

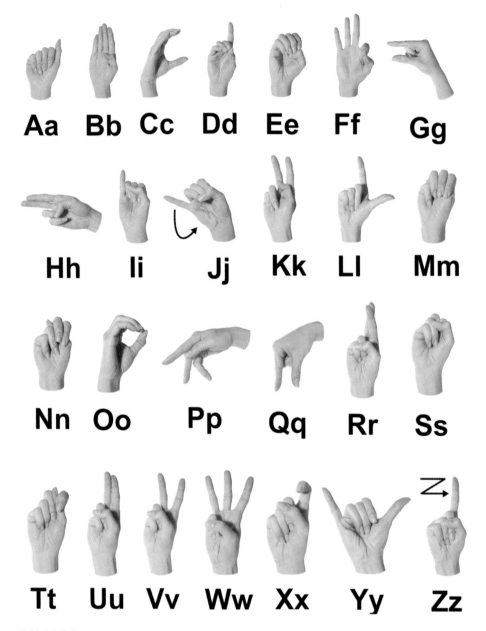

■ FIGURE 7-1

The American Sign Language Alphabet.

Source: Stephen Coburn/Shutterstock.

- **Speak slowly and articulate your words:** Many hearing-impaired patients utilize lipreading while communicating. Maintaining eye contact, speaking at a slower-than-normal rate, and properly articulating the words spoken will help to facilitate communication.
- **Utilize writing to communicate:** If a patient is unable to have an interpreter present, writing information on a tablet or small whiteboard can be an effective form of communication.

Placing the patient's needs as the main priority, careful communication, and use of the tips mentioned will help the medical assistant remain a symbol of professionalism with the hearing-impaired patient population.

Communicating with an Emotional Patient

Working with and handling an emotional patient is a skill that is developed over time and through experience. Common emotions that are dealt with in the medical office include extreme sadness, anxiety, and anger. Patients can become emotionally charged for a number of reasons. Some patients will come into the medical office visibly unstable emotionally, while others will become emotionally unstable during their office visit. It is imperative that as the medical assistant strives to develop a sensitive and professional approach to handling an emotional patient all judgment and stereotyping be cast aside.

Comforting a Sad Patient

More often than not, it is the business of medicine to cure the sick rather than maintain the healthy. It goes without saying that many patients, while in the medical office, will be given bad news as it relates to their health. Simply hearing grim news will be an emotional trigger for patients. Other times, patients will come to the medical office dealing with major life stressors: the loss of a job, the loss of a loved one, or family disruptions. Keep the following list of suggestions in mind when working with a patient who is visibly upset:

- **Maintain boundaries**: While it is important to be caring and compassionate, keep in mind that it is not the job of the medical assistant to act as a personal confidant. Do not ask questions that may cause the patient to become more upset or engaged in despair.
- **Stay on task and do not get distracted**: Maintaining control of the situation will help accomplish the tasks that are necessary and calm the patient as well.
- **Choose words carefully**: Do not try to placate a patient by saying overly affectionate terms such as *sweetie*, *darling*, or *honey*. Simply offer direct, consoling words and a specific form of assistance. An appropriate response would be, "I am sorry you are upset. Can I get you a drink of water before we continue?"

Above all, it is important to remain sincere in words and actions, consider the patient's well-being, and maintain control of the situation; do not get distracted.

Handling an Ill-Tempered Patient

Working with and handling an ill-tempered patient is trying, challenging, and oftentimes intimidating. Similar to sad or distressed patients, a patient may be or become angry or ill-tempered for a variety of reasons. The medical office manager should be made immediately

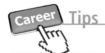

Career Tips
Continuing Education

Continuing education is a component of professionalism as it indicates that the medical assistant is keeping up to date with current medical trends, issues, and topics. Also, continuing education is a requirement for maintaining certain medical assisting credentials. Professionalism and communication have become trending topics for medical continuing education courses. In addition to learning about handling interoffice communication issues, you will find that these courses will discuss how to handle difficult and challenging patient scenarios.

aware of the situation, especially if the patient is angry about a situation that involves the medical office or a staff member. Remaining calm and not playing into the emotional drama that is caused by an angry patient should help subdue the patient. Refer to Chapter 4 for additional details regarding handling an angry patient.

Professionalism in Written Communication

Chapter 5 discussed the importance of professionalism as it pertained to the medical record, including the aspect of written communication within the medical record. Written communication extends beyond the medical record and it is necessary to discuss the professional approach that must be taken with such communication. Forms of written communication that are prevalent in the medical office include physician correspondence, patient letters, and emails among staff and other medical professionals. Personal impressions, also discussed in Chapter 6, are formed when written correspondence is received. Spelling and grammatical errors, rambling or inconsistent thoughts, and the overall visual impression of the document will cause one to form a personal impression of the sender's professionalism.

Letters

In medical offices, the written letter is the preferred method of communication especially as it pertains to patient care. Consultation notes and letters are often sent by one physician to another physician to discuss the medical care of mutual patients. These notes and letters, often termed **correspondence**, become a part of the patient's permanent medical record. When a physician is sending a letter to another physician, he or she will dictate the letter to a medical transcriptionist who will then **transcribe**, or write out, the letter while listening to the dictation. In smaller medical offices, the role of the medical transcriptionist may be assigned to a medical assistant. Professionally speaking, when completing the task of assisting with physician correspondence, it is important to maintain confidentiality on all patient matters that are being discussed. Also, it can be difficult to understand some words that are spoken during dictation. When there is doubt about a word or phrase, the medical assistant must always discuss the item in question with the physician. It is never appropriate to assume what is being said. Err on the side of caution and ask when in doubt. When completed, all forms of written correspondence should be double-checked for accuracy.

(A)

PEARSON PHYSICIANS GROUP
Shania McWalter, D.O.
123 Michigan Avenue, Parker Heights, IL 60610
(312) 123-1234

August 1, 20xx

Thomas Moore
123 Lee Street
Louisville, KY 40223

Dear Mr. Moore:

With the season for colds and flu fast approaching, it is time once again for flu shots. Supplies have arrived and flu shots will be administered starting October 3. Please call the office to schedule a visit for your flu shot at your earliest convenience.

If you wish to wait to get your flu shot at the time of your next appointment, it is not necessary to call the office. An appointment card with the date and time of your next appointment is enclosed.

Sincerely,

Shania McWalter, D.O.

ENC: Appointment card
c: B. Reed, Office Manager

(B)

PEARSON PHYSICIANS GROUP
Shania McWalter, D.O.
123 Michigan Avenue, Parker Heights, IL 60610
(312) 123-1234

August 1, 20xx

Thomas Moore
123 Lee Street
Louisville, KY 40223

Dear Mr. Moore:

With the season for colds and flu fast approaching, it is time once again for flu shots. Supplies have arrived and flu shots will be administered starting October 3. Please call the office to schedule a visit for your flu shot at your earliest convenience.

If you wish to wait to get your flu shot at the time of your next appointment, it is not necessary to call the office. An appointment card with the date and time of your next appointment is enclosed.

Sincerely,

Shania McWalter, D.O.

ENC: Appointment card
c: B. Reed, Office Manager

(C)

PEARSON PHYSICIANS GROUP
Shania McWalter, D.O.
123 Michigan Avenue, Parker Heights, IL 60610
(312) 123-1234

August 1, 20xx

Thomas Moore
123 Lee Street
Louisville, KY 40223

Dear Mr. Moore:

    With the season for colds and flu fast approaching, it is time once again for flu shots. Supplies have arrived and flu shots will be administered starting October 3. Please call the office to schedule a visit for your flu shot at your earliest convenience.

    If you wish to wait to get your flu shot at the time of your next appointment, it is not necessary to call the office. An appointment card with the date and time of your next appointment is enclosed.

Sincerely,

Shania McWalter, D.O.

ENC: Appointment card
c: B. Reed, Office Manager

(D)

PEARSON PHYSICIANS GROUP
Shania McWalter, D.O.
123 Michigan Avenue, Parker Heights, IL 60610
(312) 123-1234

August 1, 20xx

Thomas Moore
123 Lee Street
Louisville, KY 40223

RE: FLU SHOT

With the season for colds and flu fast approaching, it is time once again for flu shots. Supplies have arrived and flu shots will be administered starting October 3. Please call the office to schedule a visit for your flu shot at your earliest convenience.

If you wish to wait to get your flu shot at the time of your next appointment, it is not necessary to call the office. An appointment card with the date and time of your next appointment is enclosed.

Shania McWalter, D.O.

ENC: Appointment card
c: B. Reed, Office Manager

■ **FIGURE 7-2**

Examples of four letter formats: (A) simplified letter style; (B) modified block style; (C) modified block style with indented paragraphs; and (D) block style.

■ TABLE 7-2 **Components of a Business Letter**

Heading	The heading contains the name of the physician or practice along with the address, telephone number, fax number, and Web site address. Oftentimes, these are components of professional letterhead.
Date	Every letter should use the current date. Do not abbreviate the month or use a numerical format. Rather, write out the date, for example, January 13, 2013.
Inside address	This contains the name, title, company name, and address of the person(s) receiving the correspondence (typed four to six lines below the date).
Salutation	This is the greeting of the letter, for example, Dear Dr. Simpson (typed two lines below the inside address).
Body	The purpose of the letter is written within the body (typed two lines below the salutation).
Closing	Courtesy words such as *Sincerely* or *Kindest Regards* are included in the closing (typed two lines below the closing of the body of the letter).
Signature line	Contains the name and title of the writer. A handwritten signature is written between the closing and the signature line (typed four lines below the closing).
Reference initials	These indicate the initials of the person who typed the letter. These are found in the lower left margin in lowercase letters.
Enclosure notation	If documents are included along with the letter, the abbreviation ENC or the word *Enclosure* is written. The items in the enclosure should be numbered and listed. For example, Enclosures (2) X-ray lumbar spine Blood work dated 10/05/2012
Copy notation	When the letter is sent to another party besides the addresse, a notion is made at the end of the letter that indicates who received the copy. This is written by typing c: and the person's name. For example, c: Jane Stillman, MD

Additionally, letters will be sent to patients on behalf of the medical office. Letters of such nature may include a new patient welcome letter, a letter regarding a missed appointment, or a letter informing the patient of an overdue account balance. All letters sent to patients should be clear, direct, and to the point. The purpose of the letter should be clearly stated within the first paragraph, after the greeting. If the patient is being asked to take a specific action, such as make a payment on an overdue account, clearly state the terms and deadline for the action in the letter.

FORMATTING AND PROOFREADING With written communication, the aspect of professionalism will be taken into consideration when the recipient reviews the letter. The overall visual style of the letter as well as the terms and phrases used to express thoughts will help to convey a high level of professionalism. ■ Figure 7-2 displays various styles of letter formatting. The standard components that make up a business letter for professional communication are discussed in ■ Table 7-2.

Proofreading is essential to written communication. Word-processing software includes spelling and grammar checks; however, these functions are not necessarily helpful when medical terminology is being used. Dictionaries, thesauruses, and medical dictionaries should be readily available when writing letters.

EMAILS Medical offices will have an email address set for their staff. Many times, if the medical office has a Web site, the email addresses of staff members will be a combination of the staff member's name and the medical office's Web site domain name. For example, if Jeff Donnell is a medical assistant at Pearson Physicians Group, his email address could possibly read as jdonnell@pearsonphysiciansgroup.com. Email addresses that are assigned for work should be used solely for professional purposes and never for personal use. To do otherwise would be unprofessional.

Unfortunately, email is a mode of communication that often becomes laden with spam and forwarded chain letters, poems, and pictures. Although this type of email sharing might be amusing to some, it should never occur with work-related email accounts. Not only is this type of email a waste of time, but often such emails come with attachments that often are the gateway for malicious computer viruses. The following list will help maintain professionalism within the realms of emailing at the workplace:

- All work-related, professional emails should be formatted like a written business letter. Include closing and signature lines with email communications.
- Do not use slang commonly used for personal emails or text messaging such as LOL (laugh out loud), BTW (by the way), RU (are you), TY (thank you), or other slang abbreviations. This is not an acceptable practice when communicating professionally.
- Do not open email from individuals whom you do not know or any messages that may appear to be spam related. These can contain viruses that threaten the computer networking system.
- Respect your coworkers and peers by not using foul language or sending questionable material. Professional emails should remain conservative in nature.
- Attempt to respond to all emails that include requests for information or require direct responses within a timely manner. A good rule is to try to make all necessary replies within twenty-four hours.

As patients become more comfortable with technology and how it relates to their medical information, many will opt to send questions and concerns via email. In such circumstances, when patients are provided with staff email addresses, it is essential that there is a protocol of policies and procedures that outline what topics are considered acceptable relating to patient emailing. If there is doubt about specific correspondence and its appropriateness, seek help from the office manager.

END OF CHAPTER REVIEW

LEARNING OBJECTIVE REVIEW

Complete each learning objective to the best of your ability.

1. Explain how communication barriers can affect the role of professionalism in the medical office.

   _____

   _____

   _____

   _____

   _____

2. Describe tools that are available to assist with patients who have a language barrier.

   _____

   _____

   _____

   _____

   _____

3. List particular considerations that should be taken into account when communicating with visually and hearing-impaired patients.

   _____

   _____

   _____

   _____

   _____

4. Identify at least three top priorities when handling an emotional patient, and why they are important.

   _____

   _____

   _____

   _____

   _____

5. Name two roles professionalism plays when dealing with written correspondence.

_____

_____

_____

_____

_____

6. Summarize rules for email usage in the medical office.

_____

_____

_____

_____

_____

KEY TERMS

Use each of the following key terms in a sentence that demonstrates your understanding of the word.

1. active descriptions:_____

_____

2. barrier:_____

_____

3. bilingual:_____

_____

4. correspondence:_____

_____

5. decorum:_____

_____

6. intricacies:_____

_____

7. refugee:_____

_____

8. transcribe:_____

_____

CRITICAL THINKING

Reread the workplace scenario at the beginning of the chapter and answer the following questions.

1. What precautions should a medical office have in place to help assist patients who require translators? How could this situation have been avoided?

   _____

   _____

   _____

   _____

2. It is obvious to Talisha that the interpreter is not coming to the appointment. She must think quickly in order to help the patient and keep Dr. McWalters's schedule running as smoothly as possible. What are some tools Talisha can use to communicate with Mrs. Oktenburg?

   _____

   _____

   _____

   _____

3. When Talisha enters the exam room, she notices that Mrs. Oktenburg is visibly frustrated and upset. She has tears rolling down her cheeks. How should Talisha proceed?

   _____

   _____

   _____

   _____

DO IT YOURSELF!

Complete the modules below to demonstrate your understanding of the chapter.

Module A

Use an Internet site, such as www.wordlingo.com or www.translate.google.com, to translate the following phrases from English to Spanish. If you live in an area with a large population group that speaks a different language, translate the phrases into that population's native language.

English Phrase	Translated Phrase
Hello, my name is	
Why are you visiting the office today?	
Are you in pain?	
Is there anything else you need?	
Do you have any questions?	
Thank you.	
Have a nice day.	

Module B

With a partner, role-play the roles of a medical assistant and patients with special needs. Utilize active descriptions to help with the visually impaired patient and spell out words for the hearing-impaired patient using the American Sign Language alphabet.

Scenarios for working with the visually impaired patient:

1. The medical assistant must orient the patient to take a seat on a chair in the examination room.

2. The medical assistant must perform phlebotomy.

3. The medical assistant needs to prepare and situate a patient for stitches on his or her right leg.

Scenarios for working with the hearing-impaired patient:

1. The medical assistant is informing the patient that he or she must take two tablets of medication every day. (An aspirin bottle can be used as a prop.)

2. The medical assistant is asking the patient to point to where the pain is located.

3. The medical assistant is thanking the patient at the end of the visit.

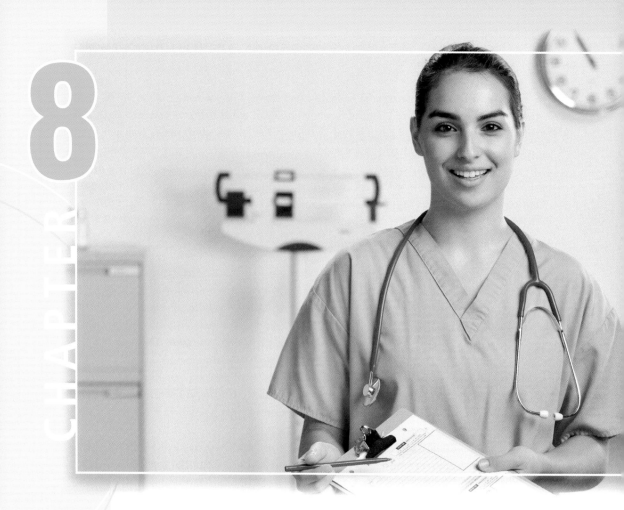

Professionalism through Emergency Preparedness

LEARNING OBJECTIVES

- Describe how knowledge, training, and proactive measures create a level of professionalism among medical assistants.

- Identify and explain three main categories of disasters.

- Explain the difference between classroom, on-the-job, and Internet-based trainings regarding emergency preparedness.

- Define two of the three specific ways a medical assistant can take proactive measures in regard to emergency preparedness.

Workplace Scenario

Carlos Cruz was recently hired to work for a small medical office in Tulsa, Oklahoma. The staff at the medical office includes a medical office manager, two administrative medical assistants, two clinical medical assistants, a physician, and a nurse practitioner. Carlos has been training at the office for two weeks and the topic of emergency preparedness has not arisen yet.

Introduction

Businesses across the United States and around the world have become acutely aware of the importance of **emergency preparedness**. Emergency preparedness is exactly what its name implies, being ready for any type of emergency at any given time. Preparedness includes everything from emergency evacuation plans to written policies and procedures pertaining to the detailed jobs and responsibilities of personnel during specific disasters.

The medical assistant will display professionalism in emergency preparedness through knowledge, training, and proactive measures. These areas are discussed throughout the chapter.

Professionalism through Knowledge

Sir Francis Bacon, an English author and philosopher, is quoted as saying "Knowledge is power." His correlation between knowledge and power is never as true or necessary as it relates to emergency preparedness. In the midst of emergency, victims feel powerless, terrified, and desperate for help. Thus, medical assistants who have acquired a firm knowledge base of the trends and strategies to cope with disasters will display their professionalism through both competence and character: competence as they correctly and knowingly assist in handling a situation, and character as they instill confidence and hope in those around them during a crisis.

Building a Knowledge Base

A firm understanding of the types of emergencies is necessary when learning how to prepare. There are three major emergencies: medical emergencies, natural disasters, and man-made disasters. Each emergency classification requires separate and specific action plans and procedures to handle given situations.

MEDICAL EMERGENCIES **Medical emergencies** are life-threatening situations such as cardiac arrest, uncontrolled bleeding, severe allergic reactions, excessive burns, and poisoning. Often medical emergencies can be the result of natural or man-made disasters. However, medical emergencies can occur at any given time and can affect a single person or multiple individuals.

The role of the medical assistant varies depending on the policies and procedures of the medical office. Nearly every medical office requires their staff members to be trained in first aid and cardiopulmonary resuscitation (CPR). Additionally, many medical offices have an emergency crash cart that is stocked with first aid items and medications. The obvious advantage available in the medical office is the direction and supervision of physicians. Most chains of command, as they relate to emergencies in the medical office, will place the physician in the highest position within the office. The medical assistant's duties during medical emergencies would likely include assisting the physician with any needs that may arise during the emergency and contacting emergency personnel. Medical assistants may also be directed to provide emergency personnel with information on circumstances surrounding the situation, any aid that has been administered, the patient's health history, and current medication list.

The medical assistant will demonstrate professionalism through individual proactive measures. Such measures would include keeping the emergency crash cart supplied and stocked with nonexpired items and ensuring their individual first aid and CPR trainings are current and up to date.

A **pandemic emergency** is another component of medical emergencies. Pandemic emergencies are classified as rapidly spreading outbreaks of disease that infects a large number of people within a specified geographical area. Geographical areas can vary from an affected county to an affected nation. The United States has dealt with various threats of pandemic outbreaks including the bird flu in 2005 and the swine flu in 2009. Every year, parts of the nation stand guard against the general strains of influenza.

Preparedness is the main component of professionally handling a pandemic outbreak. Because pandemics are specific to the disease at hand, consider the following rules when making preparations for pandemic outbreaks:

* Create a separate emergency supply kit for pandemic outbreaks. The kit should include plenty of masks, examination gloves, biohazard trash bags, syringes and needles for vaccinations, bandages, over-the-counter nonsteroidal anti-inflammatory drugs, water, and electrolyte replenishment drinks.
* Review the contents of the pandemic emergency kit on a yearly basis to ensure that its contents have not expired.
* Have the telephone numbers and Web site information available for local health departments, state health departments, as well as the Centers for Disease Control and Prevention.
* During times of pandemic outbreak, stay alert to treatment guidelines and updates as they become available from government agencies and always make mandatory reporting of infectious disease to the proper authorities when required to do so.

NATURAL DISASTERS **Natural disasters** are emergency situations that result from circumstances in nature. Common types of natural disasters include the following:

* Earthquakes
* Tornados
* Fire and wildfires
* Hurricanes and tsunamis
* Landslides
* Drought
* Winter storms

Medical assistants should be aware of the types of natural disasters that are common in their geographical areas. Their focus and attention should be on those specific natural disasters. Information on natural disasters can be obtained from community resources such as fire and

> *"FEMA's mission is to support our citizens and first responders to ensure that as a nation we work together to build, sustain, and improve our capability to prepare for, protect against, respond to, recover from, and mitigate all hazards."*

■ FIGURE 8-1

FEMA's mission statement.

Source: http://www.fema.gov/about

■ TABLE 8-1 **Government Resources for Emergency Preparedness**

Agency	Web site
Federal Emergence Management Agency	www.fema.gov and www.disasterassistance.gov
Centers for Disease Control	www.emergency.cdc.gov
Department of Homeland Security	www.dhs.gov

police departments and local Red Cross agencies. The Internet is a vast source of information. Specifically, U.S. government Web sites are exceptionally helpful. The Federal Emergency Management Agency (FEMA) is a government agency that is dedicated to helping the residents of the United States plan and prepare for disasters, as well as recover and rebuild after a disaster occurs. ■ Figure 8-1 dictates their mission statement.

■ Table 8-1 lists government agencies and their Web sites that specifically deal with emergency preparedness including natural and man-made disasters.

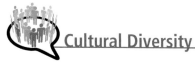 ## Cultural Diversity

It is unfortunate that since the 9/11 terrorist attacks on the United States, many Americans have negatively stereotyped individuals of Middle Eastern descent as well as those of Islamic faiths. It is necessary to recognize that these stereotypes are not only unprofessional but also hurtful and wrong. They are based on misconceptions and a lack of understanding. In the medical field, you will encounter individuals of all races, cultures, and religious creeds. All stereotypes must be ignored because everyone deserves courtesy, respect, and the best care available.

MAN-MADE DISASTERS It is unfortunate that **man-made disasters** such as terrorism, bioterrorism, industrial hazards, structural collapse, and workplace violence occur, as these are the ones that are most easily prevented. ■ Table 8-2 gives a brief description of such common man-made disasters.

■ TABLE 8-2 **Man-made Disasters**

Disaster	Forms of Implementation	Examples
Terrorism	Nuclear weapons, explosive devices, radioactive or "dirty bombs."	The attacks on the United States on September 11, 2001, raised public awareness of terrorism.
Bioterrorism	Bacteria, viruses, or toxins used to contaminate air, food and water systems, animals, and even people.	In the weeks following September 11, 2001, letters containing anthrax were mailed to individuals at media news outlets and government officials.[a]
Industrial hazards	Generally accidental in nature; could involve nuclear reactors or hazardous waste materials.	In March 2011, Fukushima, Japan, experienced major earthquakes that caused damage to the nuclear reactor in the town. More than 170,000 people were evacuated from their homes.[b]
Structural collapse	The collapse of major structures such as buildings, roofs, and bridges. The collapse may be due to faulty engineering, natural disasters, or accidents.	In 2007 a faulty beam allegedly lead to the collapse of a bridge over the Mississippi River in Minneapolis, Minnesota.[c]
Workplace violence	Violent attacks occurring at workplaces as the result of disgruntled employees and ex-employees.	In 2003, seven people were killed when an angry ex-employee of an auto parts company went on a violent rampage in Chicago, Illinois.[d]

[a]http://wwwnc.cdc.gov/eid/article/8/10/02-0353_article.htm

[b]http://theenergycollective.com/barrybrook/53461/fukushima-nuclear-accident-simple-and-accurate-explanation

[c]http://www.startribune.com/local/south/41833082.html?refer=y

[d]http://www.cbsnews.com/2100-201_162-570552.html

Professionalism through Training

Emergency preparedness training will add a tangible component to the medical assistant's knowledge base. Once the medical assistant has learned how to identify and classify emergencies, hands-on training should be completed to provide real-life situations that will require individuals to demonstrate critical thinking and action-based problem solving.

Training can be obtained in the classroom, on-the-job, or through credible Web sites.

Classroom Training

Medical assistants will begin their training for emergency preparedness in the classroom. Most medical assisting textbooks include chapters and components dealing with emergency preparedness. In addition to first aid training and CPR, learning institutions have recently begun to initiate more in-depth approaches to emergency preparedness. Students in today's classroom will learn about creating emergency kits, developing evacuation plans, creating emergency plan role-delineation charts, and **mock environmental exposure** plans. Mock environmental exposures are staged scenarios that enact the circumstances surrounding plausible emergencies.

Professionally speaking, the medical assistant's most important role will be learning to react rationally in situations and quickly assign priorities in the midst of crisis.

On-the-Job Training

Hospitals, laboratories, medical facilities, and doctor's offices are common sources of employment for medical assistants. Larger institutions such as hospitals and medical facilities will often hire professionals who specialize in emergency preparedness and prevention and risk management. Some of their typical professional titles may be director of emergency preparedness, preparedness operations specialist, or emergency preparedness planner. These individuals are generally in charge of planning and implementing all things related to emergency preparedness for the entire hospital or facility. Medical assistants working at such facilities will likely receive on-the-job training in emergency preparedness through workshops or conferences that focus on planning, preventing, and handling emergency situations. Additionally, these larger institutions may also offer programs that are available to the community and general public regarding disaster and emergency planning.

Individually owned physician practices and smaller businesses within the medical sector will often offer paid-training to their employees after business hours. Many times, it is the responsibility of the medical office manager to arrange these events. Some may choose to bring a speaker or trainer to the office and provide training on-site, while others may choose to send employees to programs and workshops within the community, paying for the cost of the program as well as paying the employees their hourly wages for attending.

Unfortunately, some offices and practices do not place importance on emergency preparedness. In such situations, the medical assistant should take initiative and speak with the office manager about the importance of preparedness. This is discussed in more detail later in the chapter.

Internet-Based Training

Again, it is important to note that recognizing the importance of emergency preparedness is a trait of a professionally minded medical assistant. If the medical assistant has not had much classroom training, and on-the-job training is lacking or nonexistent, the medical assistant should pursue other avenues in order to become adequately trained and prepared for emergencies. One of the best resources available to the medical assistant is the Internet.

Some organizations will offer courses for free, while others will charge a nominal amount. Medical assistants interested in self-training can search the Internet for **webinars**, which are online seminars that allow the participant to watch a live video feed of a presentation. Additionally, they can search for workshops and conferences around the United States. The Career Tips feature in this chapter discusses the importance of using reputable Web sites.

Career Tips

When utilizing online resources for training and educational purposes, make sure to use reputable Web sites that are being utilized are reputable. Some great starting points for finding online training and resources pertaining to emergency preparedness include government Web sites, which are indicated with "dot gov" (.gov). Additionally, well-known and recognized organizations such as the American Red Cross provide wonderful reference. Stay away from wiki Web sites such as Wikipedia. The integrity of these Web sites is uncertain as anyone can log in and alter the Web page content.

Professionalism through Proactive Measures

Proactive measures are things that are done or accomplished in order to prevent or lessen the severity of a circumstance. As a medical assistant continues to search for professional approaches to emergency preparedness, proactive measures should top the list. This chapter has already discussed possible proactive measures, including initiating an emergency preparedness plan if one is non-existent. However, more can be done by medical assistants in both their professional and personal lives.

Leading by Example

Medical assistants often live their roles as educated, compassionate, and professional individuals both at the workplace and outside of the workplace. While it is necessary to be able to separate work from personal life, the role of emergency preparedness is one example where both work and personal life is affected. Medical assistants should lead by example and take the initiative to create an emergency preparedness plan for their own homes and families. The following is a list of things that can be done in the home:

- Discuss the importance of emergency preparedness with family members.
- Identify safety zones and meeting places where family members should meet if they are to become separated during a disaster.
- Ensure family members are CPR certified and have a basic knowledge of first aid.
- Create emergency supply kits for home, work, and vehicles.

Emergency supply kits need to include more than just food or water. ■ Figure 8-2 provides a detailed list of items that should be included in all emergency supply kits.

Understanding Emotional Needs

Emergencies and disasters can be extremely taxing for individuals. Many people may experience the emotional struggle associated with injuries, loss of possessions, and the loss of loved ones. In addition, emergencies cause financial worries. Although the medical assistant is not trained to act as a counselor or therapist, he or she should be aware of the possible emotional challenges

Food & Water Supplies

☐ At least a three-day supply of bottled water for family members and pets
☐ Non-perishable food items such as canned fruit, canned beans, canned vegetables, canned soup, powdered milk, crackers, juices, beef jerky, and peanut butter
☐ Extra food and supplies for pets
☐ Consider food needs for certain age groups, such as infants and the elderly
☐ A can opener
☐ Plastic spoons and forks

Personal Items

☐ Extra prescription medications
☐ Extra pairs of prescription glasses
☐ Ibuprofen and acetaminophen
☐ Vitamins
☐ Toiletries: toothpaste & tooth brushes, mouth wash, soap, etc.
☐ Extra socks and shoes for all family members
☐ Long sleeve and short sleeve t-shirts for all family members
☐ Extra pairs of pants for all family members
☐ Blankets and sleeping bags
☐ Photocopies of identification cards and credit cards

First Aid Supplies

☐ Bandages of all sizes
☐ Antiseptic spray
☐ Antibacterial hand sanitizer
☐ Antibiotic ointment

Miscellaneous Items

☐ Whistle (to blow for location by emergency personnel)
☐ Flashlights with extra batteries
☐ Battery powered radio with extra batteries
☐ Large plastic and garbage bags
☐ Extra toilet paper, paper towels, and napkins
☐ Matches stored in a waterproof container
☐ Extra cash
☐ Small tools

Additional Items

☐ _____
☐ _____
☐ _____
☐ _____
☐ _____
☐ _____
☐ _____
☐ _____
☐ _____
☐ _____
☐ _____
☐ _____
☐ _____

■ FIGURE 8-2

Emergency supply checklist.

faced by those afflicted by tragedy. It would be wise for the medical assistant to learn about such matters through magazines, journals, and Internet articles. Also, it is possible that workshops and seminars regarding emergency preparedness would touch on these sensitive matters.

Taking Initiative on the Job

As mentioned earlier, some medical offices may not have the desire or the time to create an emergency preparedness plan. If this is the case, the medical assistant should request a private meeting with the office manager and clearly state the importance of having an emergency preparedness plan for the office. The tone of the meeting should remain respectful and non-judgmental (regarding the lack of an emergency plan), while stating the benefits of having a plan in place. It is possible the medical assistant would be assigned the task of developing the emergency preparedness plan for the office. Although some would shy away from such a task, the professional medical assistant will recognize its importance and tackle the challenge with enthusiasm.

END OF CHAPTER REVIEW

LEARNING OBJECTIVE REVIEW

Complete each learning objective to the best of your ability.

1. Describe how knowledge, training, and proactive measures create a level of professionalism among medical assistants.

   _____

   _____

   _____

   _____

2. Identify and explain three main categories of disasters.

   _____

   _____

   _____

   _____

3. Explain the difference between classroom, on-the-job, and Internet-based trainings regarding emergency preparedness.

   _____

   _____

   _____

   _____

4. Define two of the three specific ways a medical assistant can take proactive measures in regard to emergency preparedness.

   _____

   _____

   _____

   _____

KEY TERMS

Use each of the following key terms in a sentence that demonstrates your understanding of the word.

1. emergency preparedness:_____

   _____

2. man-made disasters:_____

   _____

3. medical emergencies:_____

   _____

4. mock environmental exposure:_____

   _____

5. natural disasters:_____

   _____

6. pandemic emergency:_____

   _____

7. proactive measures:_____

   _____

8. webinars:_____

   _____

CRITICAL THINKING

Reread the workplace scenario at the beginning of the chapter and answer the following questions.

1. Carlos feels he should speak with someone regarding his lack of emergency preparedness training. He is especially concerned because the medical office is located in an area termed *Tornado Alley,* where many tornados touch down every year. Whom should Carlos speak with regarding his concerns? Using specific phrases, what should Carlos say when he is given the chance.

   _____

   _____

   _____

   _____

   _____

2. Carlos has had a successful conversation regarding emergency preparedness, and he has taken on the task of developing an emergency preparedness plan for the medical office. What are some specific plans that Carlos will need to take to establish an effective plan?

   _____

   _____

   _____

   _____

   _____

3. How can Carlos help relay information regarding emergency preparedness to the patients of the medical practice?

   _____

   _____

   _____

   _____

   _____

DO IT YOURSELF!

Complete the modules below to demonstrate your understanding of the chapter.

Module A

Create a detailed shopping list of items needed of an emergency supply kit for a medical office.

Item	Quantity Needed

Module B

Create the procedural steps for the following policy regarding tornado evacuation. Remember to include the specific duties for personnel in the office, including the physician, office manager, and medical assistant.

PEARSON PHYSICIANS GROUP

EMERGENCY PLAN: TORNADO EVACUATION

Policy Creation Date: _____

Revision Date(s): _____   **Policy Number:** _____

Authorized Approval:

_____

PURPOSE: To describe, in detail, actions to be taken by the staff members of Pearson Physicians Group in the event of a tornado.

POLICY: The following procedural steps are to be followed in the event of an emergency.

PROCEDURE: The following actions detail the steps that should be taken by the respective individuals.

1.

Introduction: *These scenarios have been created to develop both communication and an interactive learning experience between students. Students should read each scenario and act out possible resolutions to each situation. The focus of the activity is not necessarily to obtain a correct answer, but rather to collectively work together to address how to professionally handle issues that may arise in a medical office. This seems out of place.*

Patty had submitted a vacation request for time off over a month ago. When the schedule came out today, she notices she is scheduled to work the entire week of her vacation request. Upset, Patty asks to discuss the matter with the office manager, who insists the request for time off must have been lost.

_____

_____

_____

_____

_____

_____

_____

_____

_____

_____

Margo is a sixty-year-old recent graduate seeking employment. She had an interview with the office manager of a pediatrician's office. During the interview the manager, referring to her age, said, "Well, I am concerned that you aren't going to be able to keep up with the fast pace of this office."

_____

_____

_____

_____

_____

_____

_____

_____

_____

_____

Shandrice is a newly employed medical assistant (MA) at a family practice. During her thirty-day orientation period, she observes her mentor Allison inadvertently administer a PPD skin test intramuscularly rather than intradermally. When Allison realizes her error, she says, "Oh, it isn't that big of a deal," and she charts the injection as being given intradermally.

_____

_____

_____

_____

_____

_____

_____

_____

_____

Mason is working at the reception desk at Pearson Medical Group. It is an extremely busy day at the practice with one doctor out sick. Mrs. Jackson checks in for her 10:25 am appointment with Mason. Mason checks the schedule and finds that Mrs. Jackson is not scheduled until next week. Mrs. Jackson promptly shows Mason her appointment reminder card with today's date and time. She mentions that she had to take time off from work to specifically make today's appointment.

_____

_____

_____

_____

_____

_____

_____

_____

_____

Carla, an MA, is working with Talisha Evans and her five-year-old daughter. They are both being seen at the office for possible strep throat. The five-year-old girl was crying and screaming during the collection of the throat culture specimen. At the end of the procedure, the child vomited due to a sensitive gag reflex and her fear of the procedure. When Carla goes into the lab area to process the specimens, she realizes that the specimen containers were not properly labeled, and there is no way to know which specimen belongs to Talisha and which specimen belongs to her daughter.

_____

_____

_____

_____

_____

_____

_____

_____

_____

Liam, a registered medical assistant (RMA), has been working with Dr. Talrico's office for three years. Two months ago Dr. Talrico hired Koshin, who also is an RMA. Liam has noticed that Koshin is very intimidated and struggles when she speaks with Dr. Talrico. He notices that she is flustered, stammers, and fumbles over her words. Liam wants to discuss with Koshin how to better communicate with Dr. Talrico.

_____

_____

_____

_____

_____

_____

_____

_____

Mateo is an office manager for Dr. Anderson's general practice. He recently hired Angela as an administrative medical assistant. Mateo notices that Angela does not make direct eye contact with patients and also has a rather curt attitude at times. Today, he received a patient complaint about Angela.

_____

_____

_____

_____

_____

_____

_____

_____

_____

Hanna witnesses her coworker Amelia take individual bottles of water out of the medical office's emergency supply kit. When she approaches Amelia about taking the water, Amelia simply states, "No one is going to miss it. Nobody even checks the kit. It is a shame to let the water go to waste."

_____

_____

_____

_____

_____

_____

_____

_____

_____

Glossary of Terms

Active descriptions a description used to explain the patient's surrounding as well as detail procedures that are being performed.

Arrogance a lofty attitude characterized by bragging and an unnecessary sense of entitlement.

Barrier an obstacle that must be overcome.

Belligerent using foul language, or the act of being aggressive or violent.

Bilingual the ability to fluently speak more than one language.

Chain of command the ranking of authority within the office, indicating the levels of supervision.

Competence having the ability or aptitude to perform a skill.

Compliant to follow a given set of rules and regulations.

Conciseness the ability to choose proper wording that is well thought out and to the point.

Confidence positively portraying personal skills and qualities with dignity while maintaining an air of self-worth and grace.

Confidential private information not to be shared without written authorization.

Consistency it refers to a uniform manner in which documentation occurs.

Correspondence notes and letters from other healthcare providers that are a permanent part of the patient's permanent medical record.

Courtesy expressing politeness and kindness through attitudes and actions.

Cover letter a letter of introduction that accompanies a résumé.

Customer service helping patients by both meeting and exceeding the needs of the patients in the medical office.

Decorum a manner of dignity and politeness.

Defaming verbal or written words that could be considered insulting or offensive.

Distraught an emotional state of being saddened, upset, or hysterical.

Efficacy something that is efficient and effective.

Efficiency effective use of time management.

Emergency preparedness being ready for any type of an emergency at any given time.

Empathy the ability to identify and share the feelings of another person.

Ethics refers to one's moral conduct, or the way in which one practices one's moral beliefs.

Externship the component of a student's education where they learn by working in real-world settings for a predetermined amount of time. For example, a medical assistant might complete 160 hours of learning in a medical office.

Gossip needless chatter that can lead to rumors, especially regarding someone's personal life.

Health Insurance Portability and Accountability Act (HIPAA) a legislative act passed in 1996 and fully enacted in 2003, designed to improve the access and portability of medical information and to decrease waste and the abuse of health insurance.

Initiative a trait that is characterized by doing above and beyond what is expected; being resourceful and creative, and tackling issues with ingenuity without having to be told beforehand.

Intricacies details or parts of a whole project.

Legible neat, easy to read and also understand.

Litigation pertaining to the act of being sued.

Man-made disasters disasters created by humans such as terrorism, bioterrorism, industrial hazards, structural collapse, and workplace violence.

Medical emergencies life-threatening situations such as cardiac arrest, uncontrolled bleeding, severe allergic reactions, excessive burns, and poisoning.

Mentor an experienced worker chosen to work with new employees and who provides the new employee with recommendations and suggestions on ways to improve personal, professional, or competency-related behaviors.

Mock environmental exposure staged scenarios that enact the circumstances surrounding plausible emergencies.

Morals what one believes to be right, true, and honorable.

Natural disasters emergency situations such as hurricanes, floods, and tornados that result from circumstances occurring within nature.

Networking a tool used by professionals to engage with other like-minded individuals within their field of expertise to create business contacts for the purpose of working together in joint business ventures.

Office for Civil Rights (OCR) a division of the U.S. Department of Health and Human Services.

Organic found within the person.

Pandemic emergency Rapidly spreading outbreaks of disease that infects a large number of people within a specified geographical area.

Parameters a distinct set of boundaries.

Personal impression a lasting mental image that reflects a person's interactions, encounters, and overall view of an event.

Portfolio a collection of information and documents that shows the aptitude and accomplishments of the student or job candidate.

Practicum also known as externship.

Proactive measures things that are done or accomplished in order to prevent or lessen the severity of a circumstance.

Professionalism it refers to the methods of one's behavior, excelling at interactions with others, and a poised and self-assured manner in which one carries themselves.

Protocol a manner of performing a procedure.

Punctual a behavior characterized by always keeping to arranged times, as for class, appointments, and so on.

Refugee a person who seeks safety in a foreign country during distressing times in their native country.

Résumé a summary of credentials, work history, experience, training, and education.

Role model someone held in high esteem based on the way he or she lives his or her personal and professional life, often demonstrating honesty, integrity, and self-discipline.

Sexual harassment unwelcome sexual advances, requests for sexual favors, and other verbal or physical conduct of a sexual nature.

Skill set specific areas of medical assisting in which you excel and enjoy.

Staffing agency a third party who has been hired by an employer to find employees to fill certain positions.

Supervisor an individual who has taken on additional responsibilities within the office and often oversees the work of others.

Syllabus a document outlining the classroom's course-work, assignments, and expectations of the student.

Transcribe to write out.

Temp-to-hire a temporary position that has the possibility of turning into a permanent position.

Temporary job sometimes referred to as temp jobs, meaning they are only for a specific amount of time such as three to six months.

U.S. Department of Health and Human Services a U.S. agency that promotes the health and general welfare of American citizens.

U.S. Equal Employment Opportunity Commission an agency committed to preventing workplace discrimination.

Webinars online seminars that allow the participant to watch a live video feed of a presentation.

Index

Note: Page numbers followed by "*b*," "*f*," and "*t*" indicate box, figure and table respectively.